BEYOND BASIC TRAINING

FITNESS STRATEGIES FOR MEN

JON GISWOLD

PHOTOGRAPHS BY **AUGUSTUS BUTERA**

ST. MARTIN'S PRESS · NEW YORK

ALSO BY JON GISWOLD

Basic Training: A Fundamental Guide to Fitness for Men

A Note to Readers: This book is for informational purposes only. Readers are advised to consult a doctor before beginning any exercise program.

www.stmartins.com

Designed and composed by Gretchen Achilles

Library of Congress Cataloging-in-Publication Data

Giswold, Jon.

　　Beyond basic training / Jon Giswold ; photographs by Augustus Butera.—1st U.S. ed.

　　　p. cm.

　　ISBN 0-312-30755-1

　　　1. Exercise for men. 2. Physical fitness for men. I. Title.

　　GV482.5.G58

　　613.7'1'081—dc21　　　　　　　　　　　　　2003046873

First Edition: November 2003

10　9　8　7　6　5　4　3　2　1

I heard something one day by chance that hit me with an impact so profound that it seemed perfect for the beginning of this acknowledgment page of my book—Information, without a system, is chaos. This book would be chaos without the passionate enthusiasm and vision of Elizabeth Beier. She trusted me enough to assemble this book my way, and I want to thank her for the giving me the system to make it work. Michael Connor for looking after Elizabeth, and to Michael Denneny for believing in me from the start.

This project would not look the way it does without the incredible talent of Augustus Butera. He and his unbelievable staff—Vanessa Rogers, Loraine Pantic, Dan Engel, and James Warren—went beyond my expectations in achieving the images for this book. The learning curve was steep, but the landing was smooth.

A special thanks goes out to Mike Lyons of the The Lyons Group (www.lyonsgroupny.com) for his continual support. The Lyons Group provided this project with models who are not only handsome and talented but are also sincere and good-hearted. Mike has that Midas touch when it comes to recognizing fresh talent and creates limitless opportunity for the following men: Adam Scorgie, Louis Gross, Jeff Herbert, Gregory Butler, Tyler Appleby, Andrew Aponick, Ted Trullinger, Matthew Foster-Moore, Peter Gaeth, Jordan Kitchen, Lawrence Bullock, Ivan Villegas, and Nico Nelson.

Personal friends who found their way onto the page for being superb athletes and role models include: John Ferris, Savvas Giautsis, Joe Petcka, Dean Dufford, Steve Jordan, David Kang, and Adam Figueroa.

Marc Wolinsky and Barry Skovgaard for the use of their breathtaking home in Water Mill, New York, and for being my best fans. Thank you to Larry Baker for feeding the guys and taking care of us all.

Ray Murray and Geert Maartens for the use of their home in Mattituck, New York, and for Ray's artful eye.

The men and women who are more than training clients, but my friends. They inspire me each and every session: Dan and Esty Brodsky, Jonathan Brodsky, Eileen Goudge and Sandy Kenyon, Jon and Joy Santlofer, Al and Claire Zuckerman, Ed McCabe, Lynn Pell, Candice Pell, Lauren Chiamotti, Larry Luckinbill, and Lucie Arnaz. I must thank all the men and women who continue to take classes with me around the world. As the saying goes, without you I am nothing.

Special thanks go out to Giovanni Falconi and Ana Vega for making my life easier, and Enid Stubin for my voice and her steady reassurance. I am grateful every day for the day I met my literary agent and good friend Ken Roberts.

Above all else, thank you Marc Raboy for staying beside me all these years. This is for Fanny.

GOING TO THE NEXT LEVEL

What do men need? George Carlin once joked that all self-help books are bogus (of course he used a different word), that getting to the store to buy a self-help book or motivational book proved that you were motivated simply by walking to the bookstore. You're motivated enough already! Turn around and go home! There is some truth to that. By picking yourself up and looking at this book, you have proved your motivation.

What men need and what men want are two separate things. I think men need options, direction—in other words, programming. Men are typically creatures of habit; once they find something that works or fits into their lives, they stick with it. Are you one of these men? I know I am. And it is important to consider. Look directly down the barrel of fear. Our fear of something new is fear of the unknown and/or the prediction of failure. Men do not like to fail. But we need to experiment and fail in order to change. In the many letters and e-mails I have received, men constantly ask about the desire to change. "How do I get my abs leaner?" "I'd like to put on some muscle, but I've been skinny my whole life. What should I do?" and "I'd like to build up to look like the guys in your book, but I don't belong to a gym. Can I still reach that goal?" These questions are honest indications that men want to change, but they don't know how. So they stick with the same routine: the same lunch, the same partner, and the same choices. *Beyond Basic Training* is a book that will offer you options. Most misconceptions and predetermined ideas of who should be doing yoga or ball training are just that. The truth is, these techniques are for every one. It is not my goal to have you fail. I want more than anything for you to succeed. I want you to change or at least to change your attitude about alternative practices. Do not turn away! You are going to find the benefits amazing. Let me get into your head and you'll find out why.

Beyond Basic Training will take you to a new level. With the current attention on Eastern disciplines and the resurrection of some tried-and-true techniques, the exercise landscape is not only becoming more and more confusing, it could cost a week's salary to buy a book for each practice and two weeks' vacation time to try them all! *Beyond Basic Training* synthesizes all of the trends of the new century and reintroduces the reader to some of the time-tested classics.

This book is broken up into three sections. Each section is comprised of information that will help you create a better body and better sense of your possibilities.

The first section, "Strategy," will help you better understand general fitness guidelines and formulas that will give you an edge when establishing a new workout routine. A client recently suggested to me that he was completely different from anyone else, and that his behavior and stubbornness in resisting exercise was unique to him. I hated to burst his bubble, but I had to make him aware that we are all very similar to each other. Our behavior keeps us from finding success. In this section you will find some exercises that will point out who you are and what keeps you from the gold medal, the spiritual calm, the success in creating the body you desire, and the self-esteem that goes along with that reachable goal.

Each strategy offers an introductory session of exercises for foundation building, a minimalist routine for time efficiency, and intermediate-level modifications of the same exercises to advance the intensity and create impressive results. This will guarantee a wide assortment of exercises to choose from so you can find the mix of training techniques that will be most effective for you.

In the "Getting Physical: Performance" section, you'll find strategies to enhance your current regimen or help you start an exercise routine. The chapter will explain where each strategy—say, Pilates—comes from. You'll learn if tools are needed in order to practice this strategy at home (balls, mats, etc.), and you'll be given a list of what to expect. Finally, the reader will be shown, through photographs and text, how to perform each exercise in each fitness strategy.

The third section, "Integration," will help you implement new attitudes about crosstraining and the benefits of heart-rate monitoring, nutritional strategies, stress management, and how to concentrate on overall better health.

Beyond Basic Training will help you break out of the dull, familiar routine you may now find yourself in and get you excited about the many options available. Crosstraining can change your fitness profile fast, and this new direction can be your guide.

A friend of mine asked me point-blank, "What is different about this book? DO we really need to read about how to do another bicep curl?" With a sea of fitness books and videotapes on the shelf, I knew what he meant. But I sold him on the concept of stability training and why it is important. He listened and agreed that the concept of balance training is vital to improve a person's fitness level and to inspire a new and improved training technique. But more importantly, he understood the need for a clear and attainable program choice. I think that people should have the choice to exercise at home and get the results that people in the health club world are offered. *Beyond Basic Training* is perfect for someone who wants dramatic results, but has limited time, funds, and resources. This book offers you a new and refreshing way to train.

Beyond Basic Training is about balance. If I can use one word to characterize this book it would be *balance*. It's what we strive for in every aspect of our lives. The balance between right and left, right and wrong, balancing our checkbook, overwork and underachievement, our personal relationships, and even our personal behavior lie in a delicate balance.

One of the first things we learn as infants is the ability to stand. Standing on two legs separates us from the animal kingdom. Standing requires balancing! Ask anyone who has an injury or weakness due to a disorder. In order to stand upright, you have to recruit muscle from your upper body, your lower body, and your midsection. Balance equals strength. By conditioning muscle systems, you can maintain balance and live a healthy, carefree life. Sounds too easy? It is easy. As we age, we lose balance. Studies have shown that after around the ages of twenty to twenty-five, our bodies begin to deteriorate. We cannot halt this part of the aging process, but we can modify it. Adding balance to physical training helps the body perform better. That's what all the buzz is about. You may have heard it called "functional training" or "natural strength." You can build a stronger body, create a stronger machine, and keep the aging process at bay by taking good care of yourself and modifying how you train.

Gravity keeps us all on Earth, right? Just because gravity is invisible doesn't mean that it doesn't have a resistance value. It places pressure on our spines as we stand and sit. The strength of our body systems keeps us upright. A major reason to consider taking up the type of strength training this book will introduce you to is to fight the effects of gravity. As with many "trends" in fitness, this philosophy isn't an overnight sensation. Many of the techniques in the following pages have been around for years, utilized by those on the search for better training models and by elite atheletes who have long used these methods to keep in ideal condition for their sport.

My goal is to get you to train for better life *function*. Function is integrated, multiplanar movement that involves acceleration, deceleration, and stabilization. In layman's terms, to function is to start, stop, and turn. Most strength and conditioning programs involve uniplanar (**sagittal plane**) force production, better known as pushing and pulling. Very little time is dedicated to neuromuscular stabilization training, core stabilization training, and **eccentric training** in all three planes of motion (*sagittal:* forward and back; *frontal:* side to side; and *transverse:* around).

A majority of exercisers perform strength-training programs on machines that have been designed without an understanding of functional anatomy, functional biomechanics, and human movement science. Machines provide artificial stabilization and only allow isolated, uniplanar training. This form of training is effective for **hypertrophy** (building muscle) but it does very little to improve daily function or prevent injury. Several machines have recently emerged and classic cable-system machines and resistance tubing, used for many years, have been reinvented to help solve this problem.

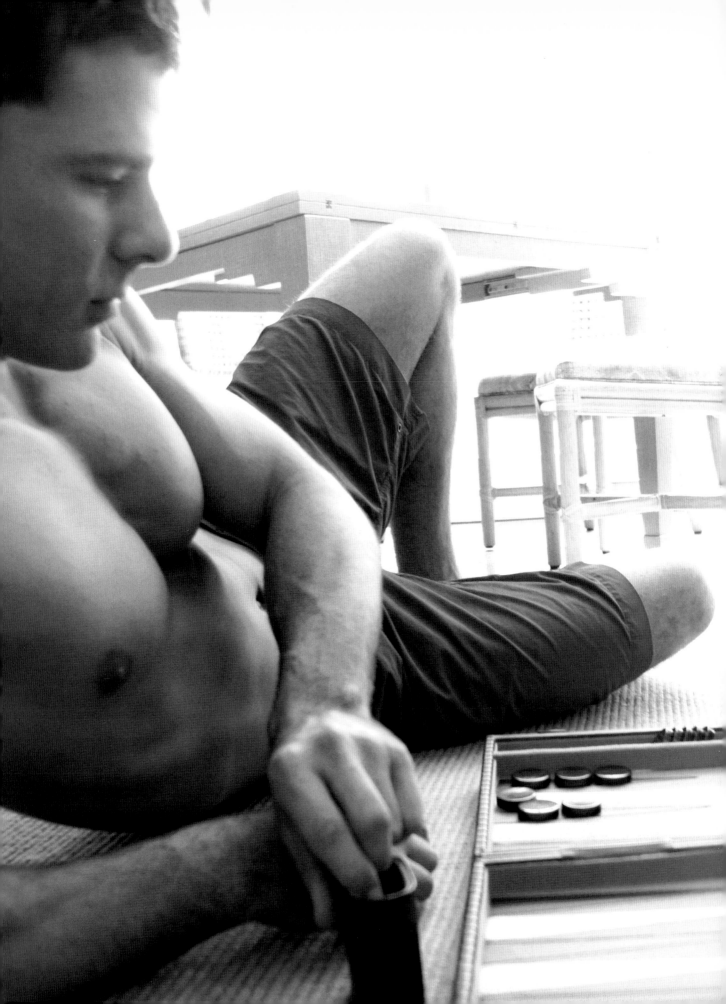

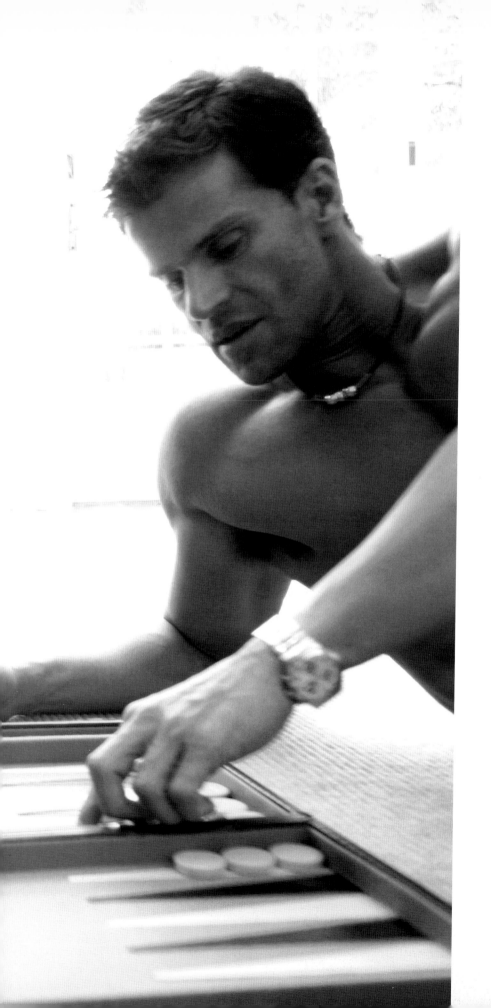

PART I

STRATEGY

(A carefully devised plan of action to achieve a goal/the art of developing or carrying out such a plan)

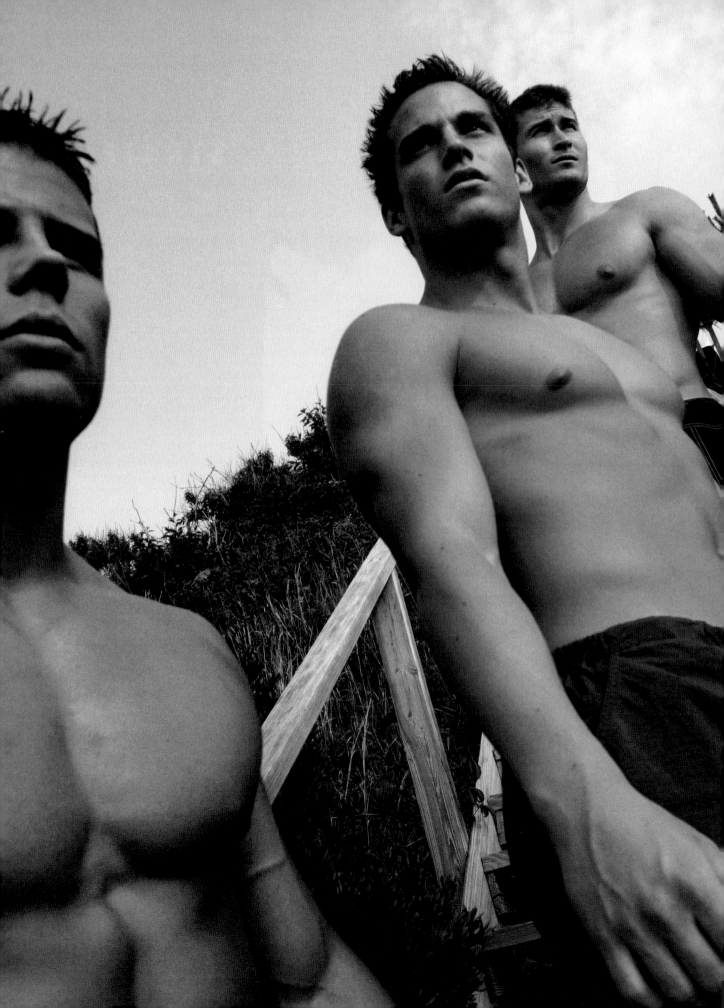

CHAPTER ONE

STRATEGY: TOOLS FOR WINNING

YOUR ROLE

Keep an open mind and allow yourself to explore the strategies introduced in this chapter. You picked up this book to look for direction. You want to be inspired. You want to see changes in your body and in your attitude. TRY.

MY ROLE

Let me be your coach. When you think of a coach who has influenced a great team or an inspirational leader, who do you think of? Why did you choose that person? What attributes does that person possess that urge people to follow him or her? I would like to be that person for you. I want you to learn something new and to find out not only how to perform exercises but how to feel better about yourself as a person. My job is to help people reach higher goals for themselves physically and emotionally.

As your coach, I want to try and bring you to a newfound appreciation of not only your body and physical ability, but of yourself as a person. My goal is to focus on *your* goals and help guide you to success by helping you understand yourself better and to identify some of the obstacles that could impede your success. I want you to find what you are looking for. That may sound simple, but the process can be filled with personal obstacles that you may be unaware of. These obstacles will always derail you unless you change the way you react toward them.

The hardest part of attempting something new is overcoming the fear of trying. After you try anything once, all you have to do from that point on is refine the task or practice until you excel at it.

TEN ELEMENTS TO CLARIFY YOUR FITNESS TRAINING PLAN.

1. **What do you want from a fit lifestyle?**

2. **Who are you right now? Describe yourself.**

3. **How do you want to train?**

4. **What are your obstacles?**

5. **How will you reach your goal?**

6. **What makes you think you can succeed?**

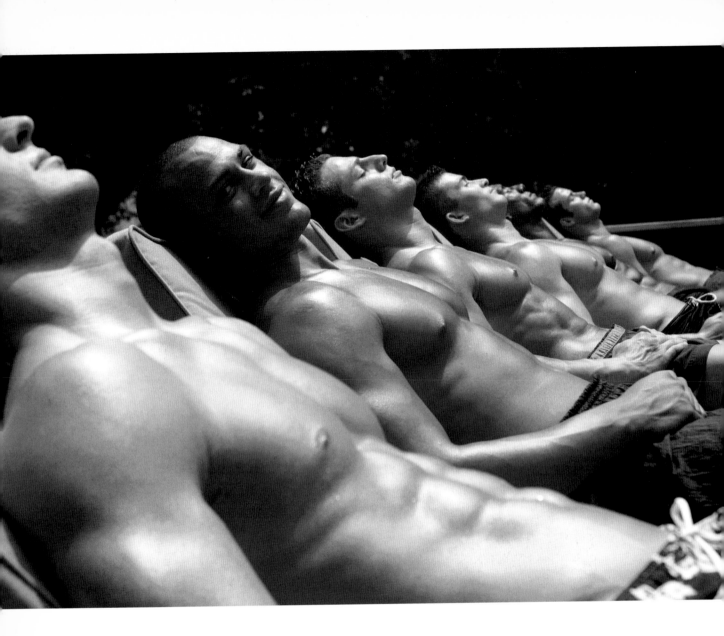

7. What technique will provide you with success?

8. What are your short-term goals?

9. What are your long-term goals?

10. Summary: What are the themes in each of the prior nine questions?

This is who you are!

CHAPTER TWO

GETTING TO KNOW YOU:

INVENTORY/SELF-EVALUATION

LIFE GAME: SELF-ESTEEM CHECKLIST

This game requires you to be honest in every true or false answer. If your answer would be "Sometimes," then answer "False" until you can honestly answer "True." If the question isn't applicable to you, then check "True."

There are fifteen questions in each category. Add up the total number of "True" checks in each section and record the figure. Add all the categories together to determine your total score.

Record your total and the date in a journal or your datebook. Compare your total to the total possible number of sixty points.

Play the game every six months until you achieve the goal of sixty points.

YOU AND YOUR ENVIRONMENT   T   F

1. My home is clean and well kept.   ☐   ☐

2. I live in a house/apartment that I love.   ☐   ☐

3. I make my bed every day.   ☐   ☐

4. I recycle.   ☐   ☐

5. I have nothing in storage that I do not need.   ☐   ☐

6. My clothing is clean, pressed, and makes me look good.   ☐   ☐

YOU AND YOUR ENVIRONMENT (CONTINUED)   T   F

7. My appliances and electrical equipment work perfectly. ☐ ☐

8. My personal papers are neat and filed away. ☐ ☐

9. My car works perfectly. ☐ ☐

10. My sink is tidy and free of dirty dishes right now. ☐ ☐

11. I have no unfinished home-repair projects. ☐ ☐

12. I live in a city/town that I love. ☐ ☐

13. My workstation is productive and inspiring. ☐ ☐

14. My refrigerator is clean. ☐ ☐

15. The food in my cupboard is fresh—not outdated. ☐ ☐

MIND AND BODY   T   F

1. I have a life beyond work. ☐ ☐

2. I floss every day. ☐ ☐

3. I have something to look forward to every day. ☐ ☐

4. I do not use illegal drugs or misuse prescriptions. ☐ ☐

5. My cholesterol is at a healthy level. ☐ ☐

6. I have had a complete physical in the past two years. ☐ ☐

7. I have no habits I find unacceptable. ☐ ☐

8. I do not smoke. ☐ ☐

9. My weight is within an ideal range. ☐ ☐

10. I am taking care of my emotional or physical problems. ☐ ☐

11. I exercise four to five times a week. ☐ ☐

12. I have my eyes tested every two years. ☐ ☐

13. I visit the dentist every year. ☐ ☐

10

MIND AND BODY (CONTINUED)

	T	F
14. I take care of my fingernails and toenails.	☐	☐
15. I limit my intake of alcohol.	☐	☐

OF THE HEART

	T	F
1. I correspond with family and friends regularly.	☐	☐
2. I do not gossip about others.	☐	☐
3. I live my life on my own terms.	☐	☐
4. I do not judge or criticize others.	☐	☐
5. There is nothing unresolved with my past relationships.	☐	☐
6. I get along with my parents.	☐	☐
7. I get along with my siblings.	☐	☐
8. I have let go of relationships that were unhealthy for me.	☐	☐
9. I always tell the truth.	☐	☐
10. I quickly clear up miscommunications if needed.	☐	☐
11. I vote and participate in the democratic process.	☐	☐
12. I have a best friend.	☐	☐
13. There is no one I avoid.	☐	☐
14. I do not make self-deprecating statements.	☐	☐
15. I am reliable and stand by my word.	☐	☐

MONEY MONEY MONEY

	T	F
1. I have no legal clouds hanging over me.	☐	☐
2. I currently live within my means.	☐	☐
3. I pay my bills on time.	☐	☐

MONEY MONEY MONEY (CONTINUED)

	T	F
4. I have paid back money that I have borrowed.	☐	☐
5. I have insurance on all my assets.	☐	☐
6. I have medical insurance.	☐	☐
7. I have a financial plan in place for the future.	☐	☐
8. All of my tax returns have been paid.	☐	☐
9. I am paid well for my work.	☐	☐
10. My will is updated.	☐	☐
11. My checkbook is balanced.	☐	☐
12. I give to charitable causes once a year.	☐	☐
13. I know how much I am worth.	☐	☐
14. I have a nest egg to fall back on in case of emergency.	☐	☐
15. My career is one that I enjoy, and it enriches my life.	☐	☐

PERSONAL GROWTH ACTIONS

Take a risk—adventure

Learn a new language—personal growth

Find a spiritual outlet—soul

Try out a new hobby—creativity

Take a sexuality workshop—sensuality

Volunteer for a good cause—humanity

Go on a date with someone new or with your significant other—relationships

ANSWER THE FOLLOWING QUESTIONS AS THEY PERTAIN TO YOU NOW, OR AT ANY TIME IN THE PAST.

History of heart problems, chest pain, or stroke?   Yes ____   No ____

History of heart problems in immediate family?   Yes ____   No ____

Increased blood pressure?   Yes ____   No ____

Increased blood cholesterol?   Yes ____   No ____

Chronic illness or special condition?   Yes ____   No ____

Difficulty with physical exercise or activity?   Yes ____   No ____

Advice from a physician not to exercise?   Yes ____   No ____

Recent surgery (last twelve months)?   Yes ____   No ____

History of breathing or lung problems?   Yes ____   No ____

Cigarette smoking habit? Number per day?   ____

Obesity (as described by your physician)?   Yes ____   No ____

Diabetes or thyroid condition?   Yes ____   No ____

Hernia or any related condition?   Yes ____   No ____

Feelings of dizziness or loss of balance?   Yes ____   No ____

Immune system disorders
(sickness, allergies, etc . . .)?   Yes ____   No ____

Any orthopedic or muscular injuries?   Yes ____   No ____

EXERCISE HISTORY AND LIFESTYLE

Please provide a full and chronological account of your exercise history that begins with your involvement or noninvolvement in high school and college athletics. Cite any and all competitive, recreational, or seasonal sport activities that have followed in your adult years and include a brief history of the various exercise programs, fitness practices, and trainers you may have also incorporated up to the present time. Highlight your age for each activity, as well as its duration and frequency.

ACTIVITY:	AGE	DURATION	FREQUENCY

Do you have any negative feelings toward, or have you had any bad experiences with physical activity or exercise?
Yes ___ No ___ (if yes, please explain)

____

Briefly describe your current physical capacity in the following areas (i.e., strong and competitive or needs improvement):

CARDIOVASCULAR ENDURANCE:

____

____

STRENGTH:

_____

_____

FLEXIBILITY:

_____

_____

SPORT SKILLS:

_____

_____

What words best describe how you view your body and its ability to perform? Why?

_____

Please list five specific things you would like to accomplish through exercise, regardless of how realistic you may be about your capacity to do so (i.e., run a five kilometer or triathlon, achieve weight loss/muscle gain, improve performance in golf or other sport, etc.).

1. _____

2. _____

3. _____

4. _____

5. _____

STRESS:

Stress takes on many forms that can be either positive or negative. Please list the predominant stress factors in your life, as they pertain to positive and negative factors.

POSITIVE STRESS FACTORS: **NEGATIVE STRESS FACTORS:**

_____   _____

_____   _____

_____   _____

_____   _____

Please identify three things you do to relieve the unmanageable stress in your life?

1. _____

2. _____

3. _____

SLEEP PATTERNS:

How many hours of sleep do you get per night? _____

Do you typically fall asleep easily? _____

What is generally the last thing you do before bedtime? _____

Do you sleep lightly or soundly? _____

How would you describe the way you feel when you wake? _____

Briefly describe your general energy level and the moods you may experience during the course of the day, citing all noticeable changes:

Morning: _____
_____

Afternoon: _____
_____

Evening: _____
_____

In the fifteen years that I have been training and teaching group exercise, I have heard many stories that have inspired me to continue on this career path. Every person comes to fitness with a history or the motive to change his or her life. Often an event forces someone to look at changing their behavior—maybe a life-threatening disease or an accident, or a sudden awareness that the scale has crept up thirty pounds since college. These realizations can be wake-up calls.

Many people look at me and the rest of the fitness community as if they were looking into a fish bowl. All of the well-groomed and carefully accessorized men who hit the gym, not to mention the growing population of personal trainers, once started where you are right now.

In 1987, I had lived in New York City for six years pursuing my version of the "making it in New York" dream. Before getting involved in fitness, I was in the fashion industry. I had been a clothing salesman since I was thirteen years old in my small hometown in northern Wisconsin and had worked my way from the Twin Cities to the Big Apple. I landed a great job at Barneys New York and, with the contacts I made, went to work selling menswear for Alexander Julian in his New York showroom. That experience led me to the idea that I could open my own design business and sell my own line of menswear. I had been designing for a few private clients and set my sights on a giant goal. This is also the time I met and started a relationship with my partner Marc. That period also introduced me to a fast-lane life of celebrities and nightlife. Small-town boy makes it in a high-profile industry in the Big City. But all of that came with a price: namely drugs and alcohol.

Then one night I discovered cocaine. It didn't take me long to become a daily user. The trouble was, I could function fairly well, or at least I thought I could. With my ego fed by a daily dose of coke and a desire to succeed in the highly competitive world of retail fashion, my addiction escalated. Isolation from most of my friends, having no nine-to-five schedule to keep, allowed me to snort more coke than work and the paranoia that comes along with that drug use set the stage for the next chain of events.

I had been on a three-day coke binge, drinking six-pack after six-pack of beer to dilute the edge of my anxiety, when I found myself sitting on the ledge of the window, on the eighth floor of the building we were living in on Nineteenth Street in Chelsea. It was the middle of the night. No sounds reached me other than the occasional cab whisking down Seventh Avenue or a distant horn. It seemed as though there was no way off that ledge other than plummeting down to the street. It seemed the right thing to do. It seemed like the *only* thing to do. But I remember having to pee. I thought that I would get up and go and pee and then jump. This is truly what was going through my mind. I didn't know how else I could stop my heart from beating so fast and my mind from spinning hopeless thoughts of inadequacy and negativity. On the outside I was the ever-optimistic Jon, but on the inside I was a drug addict—nothing more.

I climbed off the ledge to go into the bathroom and I caught a glimpse of myself in the mirror behind the dining table. I weighed less than 150 pounds, and in my underwear I looked like a concentration camp prisoner. My eyes were sunken into my forehead, dried blood crusted my nostrils from the two grams of cocaine I had consumed over the last few days. My skin was gray, and my spirit broken. I froze at the sight of myself in the mirror, and it was as if a light switched on in my soul. I cried. I thought that I had already died and this was my punishment—nonexistence. I had no feelings and no appetite to live. But in that moment I *saw* myself. I cried harder. I cried for the man I had become and for the power I had given up to drugs and booze. I cried so hard it hurt.

But hurting meant that I was still alive, alive in a way that I had not been in several months. This was my threshold. I walked through it knowing that I would have to make a dramatic change in my life in order to live. I fell asleep on the floor after writing a pledge to Marc and to myself for a new life.

The next day I went to an AA meeting. I hoped that I would find answers and people who could help me, but I was scared and alone in my own head. The room was filled with kind faces with eyes that could see directly into my bruised spirit. I sat there as quietly as I could, listening to the words and stories that seemed to make sense but that seemed so foreign at the same time. I knew it was important at least to speak my name and begin the process. I raised my hand. "Hi, my name is Jon. I am a drug addict and an alcoholic."

The next day I found myself on what they call a pink cloud. Feeling as if I had taken a giant step forward, I went to work, only to find that the space I was sharing was no longer a space I was welcome in. My papers had been packed up alongside a few boxes of sweaters and pants, sitting next to the door. I was told to find a new place to run my business. My first feeling was shame and then anger. How could this be happening when I was trying to get everything together? But it *was* happening, and the only thing I could do was grab my stuff and go.

With my boxes in tow, I went looking for a space to set up my floundering business. Somehow I trusted each step I was taking. I found a sign that said OFFICE FOR RENT on Twenty-second Street, just off Sixth Avenue, in the warehouse section of the Flatiron District (one block away from my publishing house). The office was a three-hundred-square-foot space adjacent to a printing business. I knew this office would be mine. In such a fragile state, I wasn't sure the landlord would want me as a tenant. His name was Ray, and he was a nice guy. For $350 a month, I could move in that day.

I was going to get the rest of my things and was waiting for the traffic light on Sixth Avenue to change when I heard a female voice say, "Is your name Jon?" I didn't respond. A tap on my shoulder. "Excuse me, are you Jon?" I nodded. "I heard you speak at a meeting the other night, and I was wondering how you're doing." I looked at an open face and inviting eyes and felt as though I mattered. The simplest of gestures can make a world of difference. I felt I had joined the human race again, like I had a place in it. The woman invited me to her exercise studio, which just happened to be across the street from my new office space. I agreed and stepped directly into a change that would dramatically affect my life and career. I stepped into my future.

Molly Fox Studios became a home away from home, an educational institution, a safe house and temple for many others and me. I was introduced to group exercise, which was just beginning to find its popularity in the United States. Jane Fonda was the toast of the industry, and Molly and her team of teachers were inventing new exercise methods and creating new techniques. I wanted in on this not-so-well-kept secret. My business had all but dried up. The stock market collapse of October 1987 essentially ended my design business, and I immersed myself in exercise. I took low-impact classes, body-sculpting classes, high/lo-impact, funk dance, abs classes, and stretch and tone. I could not get enough. Sometimes I took two or three classes a day. When I wasn't in class, I attended meetings. I was getting better. I was getting stronger. I was finding Jon.

I looked upon the men and women who taught Molly Fox's classes as idols. They radiated health and well-being. I knew that I wanted this to be my life. It was as if someone had tailor-made this career for me. Teaching offered everything that I wanted. It required expression, dance and movement, physical rushes and concrete results, applause, and a connection with people. There was no money in the field unless you earned it. We were paid twenty dollars an hour and one dollar a head over ten people. Today, that seems like nothing, but the first class I taught, where I had three people in my class, still remains one of the highlights of my life. I worked hard at fine-tuning my class and creating choreography, getting myself certified by fitness associations, and becoming an educator. Molly had high standards and expected the same of her staff. I was on my way. At the same time that I was finding my professional self, I was finding my *true* self. This time in my life gave me back my life. I am grateful each and every day that I work in the exercise field and can inspire others to get fit.

Molly Fox will always be my mentor and hero. I truly owe her more than thanks. She and I counted our first ninety days of sobriety together, and she invited me into a world that would have passed me by had she not tapped me on the shoulder and exercised the simplest form of humanity, an act of kindness.

GET OVER IT AND ON WITH IT

There comes a time when you have to take charge of your mind, your body, and your behavior. Whatever pushed the buttons that caused you to be defeated needs to be replaced. It's time to trade in your history for the present.

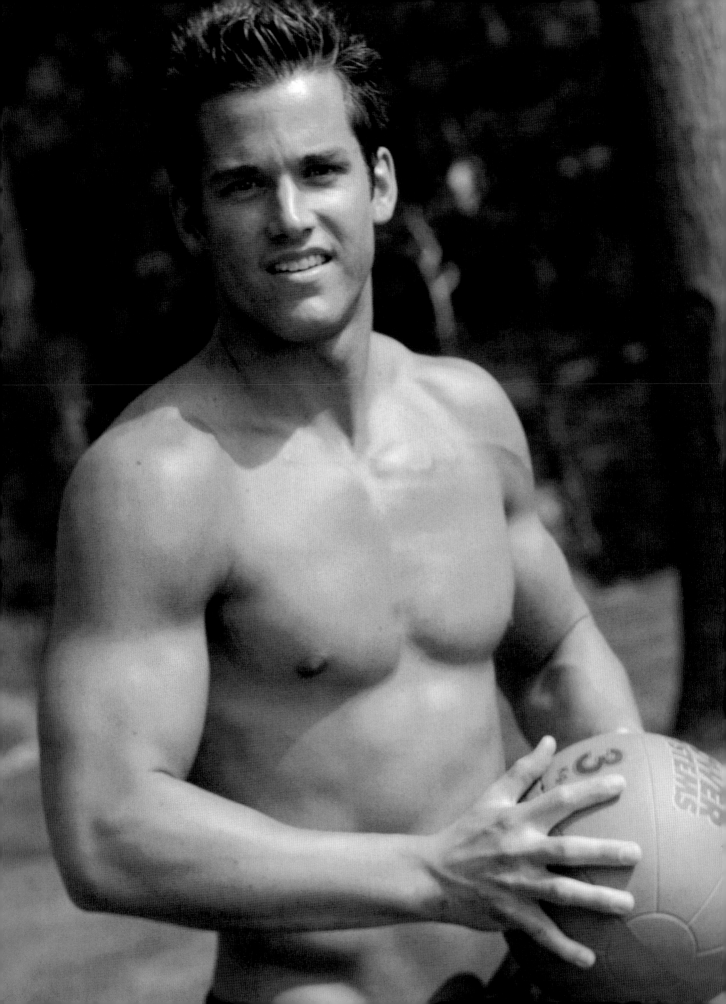

READY, SET . . . BEFORE YOU GO

Before you begin to exercise, consult with a qualified health practitioner, such as your physician. A preexercise assessment will help you determine the safest, most appropriate way to start your program.

Next, determine your short-term and long-term goals. Pursuing attainable goals will increase your self-esteem and self-confidence. Don't worry if you're feeling nervous about beginning an exercise program. Everybody does!

THE BIG THREE PLUS ONE

Your exercise program should concentrate on the following areas:

IMPROVING AEROBIC ENDURANCE. For aerobic exercise, your choices are numerous. Swimming and water exercise are excellent because they don't place a lot of stress on the joints. Stationary and seated

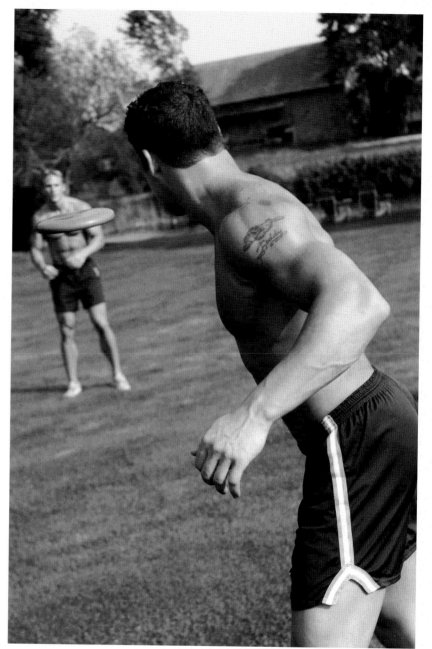

(known as recumbent) cycling are less stressful on the back and legs than some activities, and fitness walking is also a good option.

Try to follow the guidelines from the Centers for Disease Control and Prevention (CDC) and the American College of Sports Medicine (ACSM). These guidelines recommend that you accumulate forty minutes or more of moderate-intensity physical activity four or more days of the week.

INCREASING STRENGTH. Resistance training has gained considerable popularity with older adults over the last decade. It has been shown to stimulate bone growth, improve posture, decrease the percent of body fat, and improve balance and mobility. To ensure you train properly and effectively, procure the expertise of a certified personal trainer or instructor and have him or her design an appropriate resistance exercise program for you. (In fact, seeking the support of one of these professionals can help you adhere to the correct exercise safety guidelines and maximize the effectiveness of all types of exercise.)

IMPROVING FLEXIBILITY. You need to perform flexibility exercises in a slow, sustained manner, holding the stretches for up to thirty seconds. Make sure you feel the stretch in the muscles, rather than the joints. It is okay to stretch daily. Stretches for the backs of the legs, fronts of the legs, low back, and shoulders are recommended. These flexibility stretches are best performed at the end of the workout.

CORE TRAINING. The plus in our list. Core training has gained popularity, not because of the endless six-packs that grace the pages of every magazine or the rack of abs that every soap star displays, but because "core" has become the latest trend in the fitness industry. It stabilizes the low back and pelvis and works to maintain proper posture and body alignment as we move through our daily activities. Once the core has been established, there are few changes that need to be added to a regular fitness routine. The biggest change may be to start using your core to hold your body position and alignment while working out.

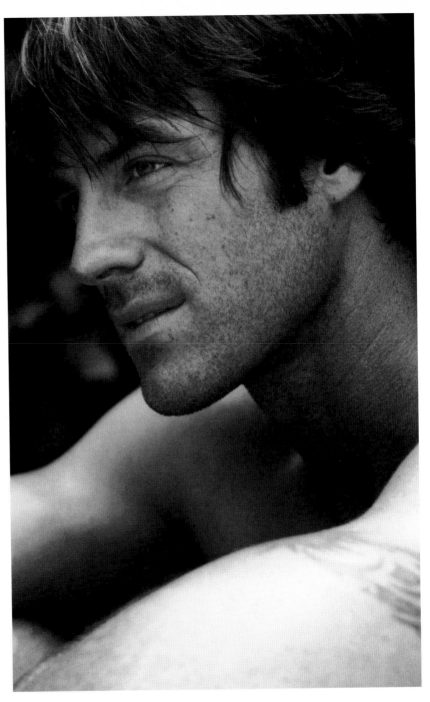

BEFORE YOU START AN EXERCISE PROGRAM, QUESTION YOURSELF

There are a few questions to ask yourself to determine whether you should see your doctor first.

Your first step is to ask yourself how active you want to be. This may sound like a silly question—you're probably planning on doing whatever you're capable of, whether that's a slow walk around the block or a vigorous step class. But if you're of a certain age or have certain cardiovascular risk factors, you may need to see your physician before beginning a program that involves vigorous (as opposed to moderate) aerobic activity.

HERE'S HOW EXERCISE INTENSITIES ARE TYPICALLY DEFINED

LOW-TO-MODERATE. This is an intensity that can be sustained relatively comfortably for a long period of time (about sixty minutes). This type of exercise typically begins slowly, progresses gradually, and usually isn't competitive in nature.

VIGOROUS. This is an intensity that is high enough to significantly raise both your heart and breathing rates and is usually performed for about twenty minutes before fatigue sets in.

Are you planning to participate in vigorous activities and are a man over forty? You should receive a medical exam first. The same is true for individuals of any age with two or more coronary artery disease risk factors (see page 24). If you're unsure if this applies to you, check with your physician.

MORE QUESTIONS

Now that you've made it through the first questions, there are a few more to answer. A "yes" to any ONE of the following questions means you should talk with your doctor, by phone or in person, BEFORE you start an exercise program. Explain which questions you answered "yes" to and the activities you are planning to pursue.

1. Have you been told you have a heart condition and should only participate in physical activity recommended by a doctor?

2. Do you feel pain (or discomfort) in your chest when you do physical activity? When you are not participating in physical activity? While at rest, do you frequently experience fast, irregular heartbeats or very slow beats?

3. Do you ever become dizzy and lose your balance, or lose consciousness? Have you fallen more than twice in the past year (no matter what the reason)?

4. Do you have a bone or joint problem that could worsen as a result of physical activity? Do you have pain in your legs or buttocks when you walk?

5. Do you take blood pressure or heart medications?

6. Do you have any cuts or wounds on your feet that don't seem to heal?

7. Have you experienced unexplained weight loss in the past six months?

8. Are you aware of any reason why you should not participate in physical activity?

If you answered no to all of these questions, you can be reasonably sure that you can safely take part in at least a moderate physical activity program. But again, if you are over forty and want to exercise more vigorously, you should check with your physician before getting started. By taking the time to evaluate whether you are ready to start exercising, you've planted yourself firmly on the path to better health and fitness.

CORONARY ARTERY DISEASE RISK FACTORS

Age (men over forty-five, women over fifty-five)

Family history of heart attack or sudden death

Current cigarette smoking

High blood pressure

High cholesterol

Diabetes

Physical inactivity

ACSM GUIDELINES FOR HEALTHY AEROBIC ACTIVITY

The American College of Sports Medicine (ACSM) recommends the following:

Exercise five times a week.

Warm up for five to ten minutes before aerobic activity.

Maintain your exercise intensity for thirty to forty-five minutes.*

Gradually decrease the intensity of your workout, then stretch to cool down during the last five to ten minutes.

FITTING IN FITNESS

One of the most popular excuses for failing to work out is not having enough time. Are you really so busy it is impossible to squeeze in exercise? Or is it more likely your time is spent on things that are not top priorities for you? If you frequently use lack of time as an excuse for missing workouts, fill in the following chart.

YOUR USE OF TIME

Being totally objective, fill out the following top-ten list with items that are most important to you, ranking them in order of importance. Think in terms of your overall life and what you love the most.

TOP TEN THINGS IN MY LIFE

1. _____

2. _____

3. _____

4. _____

5. _____

6 _____

7. _____

8. _____

9. _____

10. _____

Now list the top ten ways you currently spend your time, from the most to the least time consuming.

TOP TEN WAYS I USE MY TIME

1. _____

2. _____

3. _____

4. _____

5. _____

*If weight loss is your major goal, participate in your activity for at least forty minutes for five days each week.

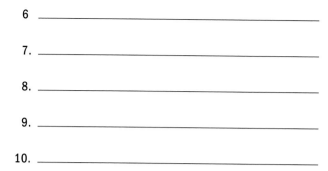

6 _____

7. _____

8. _____

9. _____

10. _____

Take a look at list 2. From that list and your experience, note any activities that whittle away at least ten minutes of your time a day. Include things like waiting in store lines, waiting on hold on the phone, being stuck in traffic, waiting for clients, watching TV, etc. Beside each entry, state how much time gets spent and add up your average daily total.

TIME I WASTE DAILY

1. _____

2. _____

3. _____

4. _____

5. _____

6 _____

7. _____

8. _____

9. _____

10. _____

TOTAL WASTED TIME EACH DAY
(HOURS/MINUTES): _____

WAYS OF INCREASING TIME FOR FITNESS

Compare list 1 with list 2. Do you devote the majority of your time to what means the most to you? Or do you find yourself using precious time on activities that really don't mean that much? If your two lists do not enhance each other, it is time to get your priorities in line. For example, if your number-one priority is enjoying your family, yet you work long, hard days to support them, you may need to look at working shorter days for less pay.

Now look at list 3. The purpose of this exercise is twofold. First, it shows we all waste time. After all, no one can be expected to run full tilt without a moment of rest. There is always time available for health and fitness; it is simply a matter of motivation. (If you won the lottery, wouldn't you find time to pick up the money?) Second, this list shows that planning your time more wisely can free up other parts of the day. For example, if you find yourself holding on the telephone a lot, use that time to pay bills or make a grocery list. While you are waiting in a doctor's office or under a hair drier, why not catch up on your work-related reading? Then you will have effortlessly saved yourself a chunk of time for exercise and other fun things.

How much do you value yourself? If you pack the day so full there is no time for you, you are stressing yourself beyond human limits. The body and mind need exercise and rest to stay fit and well. Take a closer look at your use of time to find a way to ease activity into your lifestyle.

HOW DO YOU MEASURE UP? TESTING— ONE, TWO, THREE

It seems we are all trying to get into better shape and enhancing our lives by eating healthier, cutting out or back on vices, and getting regular exercise. But how are we doing? Sure, you can fly on that new elliptical machine they just put in at the gym, but can you climb several flights of stairs if the elevator in your building is out of service?

Ask yourself:

Can you walk at a fast pace for ten minutes without feelings out of breath? = AEROBIC FITNESS

Can you run the last couple of blocks to a meeting you're running late for without collapsing? = ANAEROBIC POWER

Can you lug a full briefcase and/or a backpack around without feeling totally exhausted? = UPPER BODY STRENGTH

Can you surf the Internet without sitting hunched over your computer? = CORE STRENGTH

Can you balance on one foot to tie your sneakers? = BALANCE

Can you pick up a coin without bending your knees? = FLEXIBILITY

Does the waistband of your pants stay flat (without folding over) when you go beltless? = BODY FAT

If the answer to any of these questions is **no**, you should find out how you measure up. The following tests will provide you with a foundation for setting up a program that will boost your performance in all real-life areas, not just at the gym. You may look great from all the work lifting and running, but can you improve your performance overall in the real world, a world where you have to run after buses, lift cartons to the top shelf in your closet, sit up during an important meeting, move easily through a spirited game of volleyball, or just enjoy a good night's sleep? You will benefit by training in all areas of fitness. The body beautiful is great to look at, but a strong and capable body is even more satisfying. Don't leave a weak link in the chain, especially if you are building and training the "show me" areas.

To take the following short tests you'll need a second hand on your watch or clock, a standard chair, and a measuring tape (Yikes!). The tests are graded for a man between the ages of twenty-seven to forty-one years of age. The results for a younger man would involve a lower heart-rate count and higher repetitions in the strength test. Remember that you are only testing yourself, and the results are for your information only. How you use what you find out is up to you as well.

AEROBIC WALK. Walk for ten minutes as quickly as you can without breaking into a jog. Then take your heart rate by touching your neck next to your Adam's apple with your fingertips for ten seconds. Multiply that count by six, which equals how many times your heart beats per minute of aerobic exercise. Results vary with different ages. A score of under 90 is excellent, 90–100 is good, 100–25 is fair, over 125 needs some work.

"HOME" WORK—Walk three times per week for at least thirty minutes at about 3.5 miles per hour.

ANAEROBIC CLIMB. Walk up about forty to fifty steps without stopping. If you need to go up and

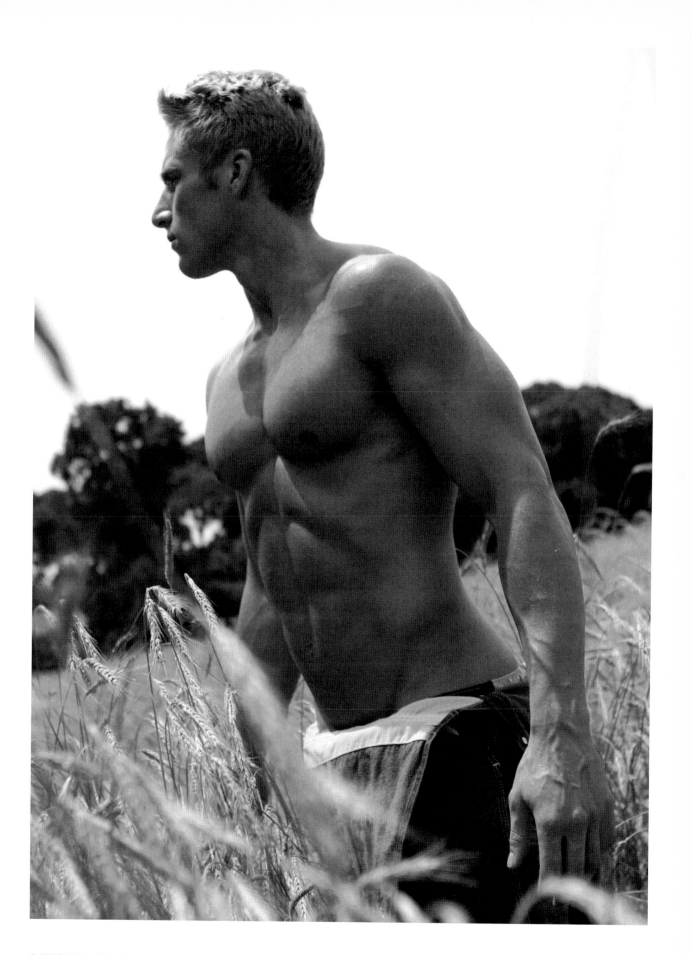

down a single flight of stairs then do so. Wait sixty seconds before you take your heart rate, as described above, on the neck for ten seconds (multiply by six). Under 90 is excellent, 90–100 is good, 100–25 is fair, and over 125 needs improvement.

UPPER BODY STRENGTH—PUSH-UPS. Hooray for the standard push-up! In the traditional push-up position, with both hands on the floor slightly wider than your shoulders and on your toes with your legs extended, count as many push-ups you can do without stopping or losing your technique. Over fifty is excellent, thirty-five to fifty is good, twenty to thirty-five is fair, and under twenty means you need to improve.

CORE STRENGTH—CRUNCHES. Lie on the floor with your knees bent and your feet flat on the floor. With your hands behind your head, curl your upper body toward your lower body enough to clear your shoulder blades off the floor. Count as many crunches as you can before you feel you have to stop. Fifty-five and over is excellent, forty to fifty five is good, twenty-five to forty is fair, and under that needs improvement.

BALANCE—ONE-FOOT STAND. You may think that knowing how to balance is obvious, but balance requires both strength and concentration. As people age, they may lose their ability to balance. Stand on your strongest leg (the same side as the side you write) with your knee slightly bent. Raise the other leg, lifting your foot about two inches off the floor while keeping your arms relaxed at your side. Try to balance for at least thirty seconds. Over thirty seconds is excellent, twenty to thirty is good, eleven to twenty is fair, and if you can only manage fewer than ten, stay away from the balance beam.

FLEXIBILITY—TOE TOUCH. Stand with your feet separated a hip-width apart, with your knees slightly bent to unlock the joints. Bend forward from the hip joint, allowing your arms to reach toward the floor until you feel a comfortable stretch. Note how close your hands come to the floor. Slowly return to a standing position. Hands flat on the floor is excellent, touching the top of your shoes is good, touching your ankles is fair, and touching your midshin requires some attention.

BODY FAT—AND THE ANGRY INCH

The cruelest test of them all. Strip. Take a look at yourself in the mirror, a good look. Trying pinching the skin away from muscle in three key areas: the chest, on the outer side between the nipple and the armpit; the waist, two inches from your belly button or the love handle area; the leg, on the inner side of the thigh. Use your index finger and thumb. If you cannot pinch any fat away from these areas, call me. If you can pinch an inch or more of fat away in any of these areas, the red flag has been raised.

> **"HOME" WORK**—Increase your cardio routine in duration or intensity and take an honest look at what you're eating.

Most health clubs and fitness centers with a staff of trainers can provide a methodical exam you can take to find out your exact measurements in a more scientific way. It is a good idea to have a formal assessment before you begin a workout routine to identify the areas that need work and to get an overall estimation of how fit you are. This test is a casual way for you to test your levels in the privacy of your own home. For those who pursue a regular fitness routine, it can also be a nice way to see progress and the results you have worked so hard for.

BATTLING BOREDOM

Do you find it difficult to get out of bed in the morning for your daily walk and easy to make up excuses to skip the gym on the way home? Even the most dedicated exercisers occasionally get bored with their routine. Waning motivation, cutting workouts short, and not feeling your old enthusiasm are all signs of a stale exercise regimen.

QUICK FIX

Evaluate your current routine to determine which part of it really bores you. A new variation on your favorite activity—such as cardiofunk or kickboxing instead of step aerobics, or hoisting free weights instead of working on machines—may be enough to reinvigorate a stale routine.

If you've always worked out indoors, logging miles on a treadmill, stairclimber, or stationary bike, move your workout outside for a change of scenery. Run, hike, or bike on trails; swim in a lake or ocean.

BIGGER CHANGES

When tweaking your routine isn't enough, make bigger changes. Take up an entirely new activity—especially something you never thought you'd do. If you've always stuck to solitary pursuits, sign up for a team sport, such as volleyball, basketball, or even doubles tennis. Or tackle something you've always shied away from—indulge your thirst for adventure with a rock-climbing class (start on an indoor wall, then move to the real thing as your skills improve).

GOOD COMPANY

Working out alone can provide an oasis of solitude in a busy day, but maybe you need some company. Exercise companions add a social element to any routine. Ask a friend to be your workout partner—you won't skip a workout if someone is waiting for you.

Just about every sport or activity has a club; to find one, ask around at gyms or local community centers. Keeping up with the crowd also means you'll be challenged to improve your skills. Ask about organized workouts and fun runs offered by local track clubs, as well as group rides hosted by cycling clubs. These

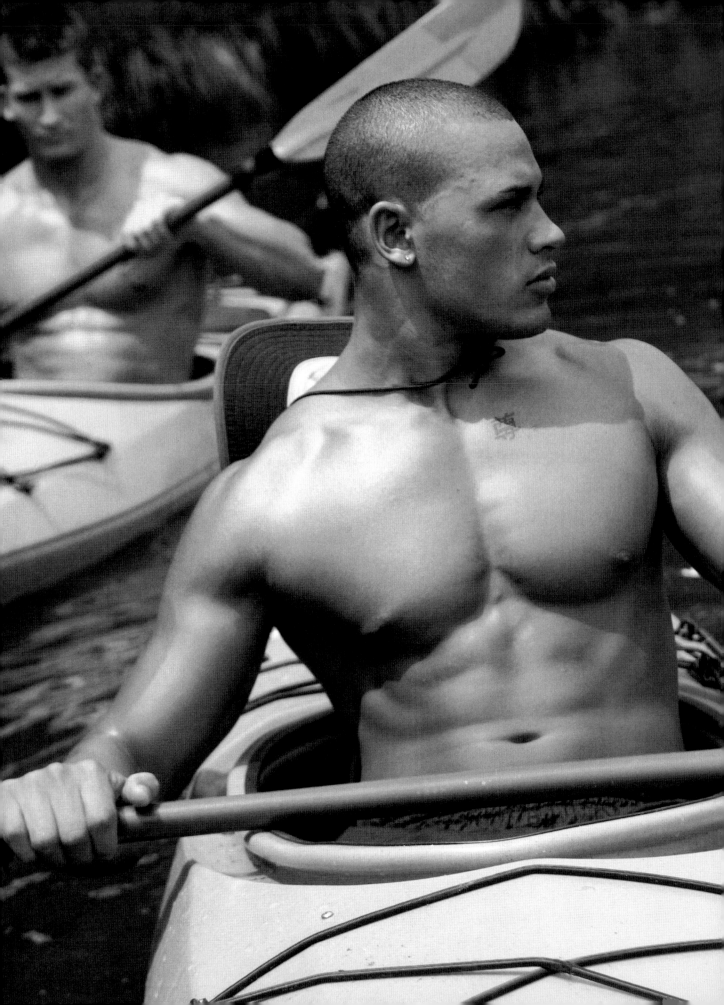

clubs also develop a community of others who share the same interest in a healthy lifestyle.

CHALLENGE YOURSELF

Many exercisers work out simply to stay in shape, and that's a worthy goal. But setting a big goal, such as finishing a ten-kilometer race or completing a rough-water swim, will give your daily workouts more meaning.

Start by incorporating bursts of speed into your workouts. After a gentle warm-up, alternate a fast pace with a slower one for recovery. This can be as simple as sprinting to the next tree or as structured as running intervals on a track or sprinting laps in the pool.

ADD VARIETY

Elite triathletes pioneered crosstraining, and it works for the rest of us, too. If you usually focus on one activity, substitute another a few days a week. Ideally, any exercise program includes elements of cardiovascular exercise, weight training, and flexibility.

NEW TOYS

Small exercise gadgets aren't necessary, but they can make your workouts more fun and challenging. Heart-rate monitors, aquatic toys, such as buoys and gloves, and safety equipment are just a few items to consider. Find out which new training gadgets are available for your favorite activity.

TAKE A BREAK

Sometimes you really do need time off. In that case, cut back on your usual routine and substitute other ac-

tivities. You might even find some that you enjoy more than your old favorites.

Once you've fought your first battle with boredom, you'll know the tricks to keep exercise from becoming too routine. Trying new sports, new classes, and new activities—and learning how to spice up old favorites—can help you overcome the inclination to devise creative excuses for not working out.

SLOWING THE AGING CLOCK

As you grow older, you may feel there is nothing you can do about the physiological changes that occur with aging. Surprise! There *is* something you can do, and it needn't even cost anything. What is it? *Exercise!*

THE AGE ANTIDOTE

Research has discovered the following in exercisers over the age of seventy.

- Physical activity in elders has been linked to the prevention of some cancers, as well as reduced risk of heart disease, hypertension, osteoporosis, obesity, Type 2 diabetes, and osteoarthritis.

- Mature adults who maintain high levels of cardiovascular endurance, strength, and flexibility are less likely to need long-term care.

- Falls, which are the leading cause of fatal injuries in people over seventy-five years old, can be reduced dramatically through participation in exercise programs that improve balance and mobility.

- Increased strength improves gait and bodily control and helps individuals function independently.

- Exercise is often associated with more effective stress

management, fewer sleep disorders, enlightened mental outlook, reduced loneliness, and lowered depression and anxiety.

HEART RATE

Your training heart-rate zone is a critical element in exercise. Taking your pulse and figuring your heart rate during a workout is one of the primary ways to ascertain the intensity level at which you and your heart are working. There are many ways to measure exercise intensity. The Karvonen Formula is one of most effective methods used to determine heart rate. Rating Perceived Exertion (RPE) and talk-test methods are subjective measurements that can be used in addition to taking a pulse.

THE KARVONEN FORMULA

This is a heart-rate reserve formula and one of the most effective methods used to calculate training heart rate. The formula factors in your resting heart rate, so first, you'll need to determine your resting heart rate by doing the following:

- Prior to getting out of bed in the morning, take your pulse on your wrist (radial pulse) or on the side of your neck (carotid pulse).

- Count the number of beats, starting with zero, for one minute. If you don't have a stop watch or a clock with a second hand in your bedroom, you can measure the time by watching the number change on a digital alarm clock. Find your pulse and start counting when the minute number changes; stop counting when it changes again.

- To help assure accuracy, take your resting heart rate three mornings in a row and average the three numbers.

The next step in finding your training heart-rate zone is determining the intensity level at which you should exercise. As a general rule, you should exercise at an intensity between 50 to 85 percent of your heart-rate reserve. Your individual level of fitness will ultimately determine where you fall within this range. Use the following table as a guide for determining the best intensity level for you:

BEGINNER OR LOW-FITNESS LEVEL	50%–60%
AVERAGE FITNESS LEVEL	60%–70%
HIGH FITNESS LEVEL	75%–85%

Once you've determined and gathered this information, pull it together with the Karvonen Formula:

220 – AGE = MAXIMUM HEART RATE; THEN

MAXIMUM HEART RATE – RESTING HEART RATE × INTENSITY + RESTING HEART RATE = TRAINING HEART RATE

For example, Eric is thirty-three years old, has a resting heart rate of seventy-five and he's just beginning his exercise program (his intensity level will be 50 to 60 percent). Eric's training heart-rate zone will be 131 to 142 beats per minute:

ERIC'S MINIMUM TRAINING HEART RATE
220 – 33 (AGE) = 187
187 ÷ 75 (RESTING HEART RATE) = 112
112 × 0.50 (MINIMUM INTENSITY) + 75 (RESTING HEART RATE) = 131 BEATS/MINUTE

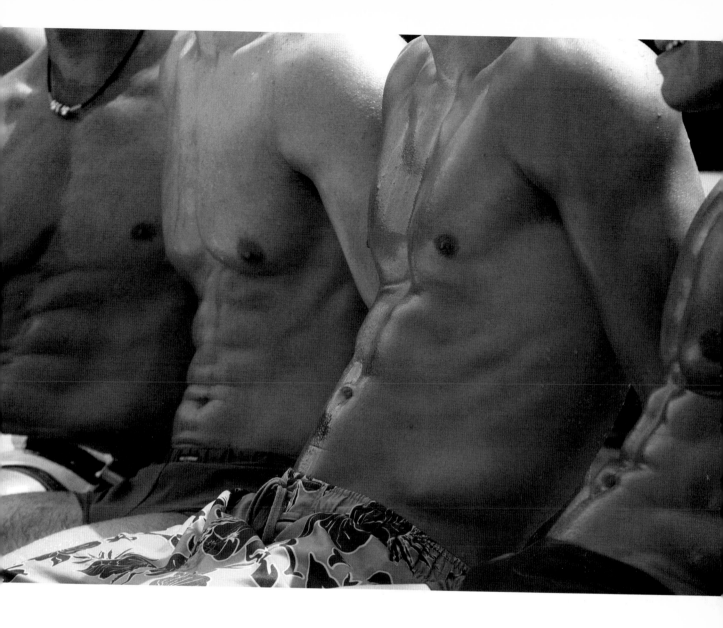

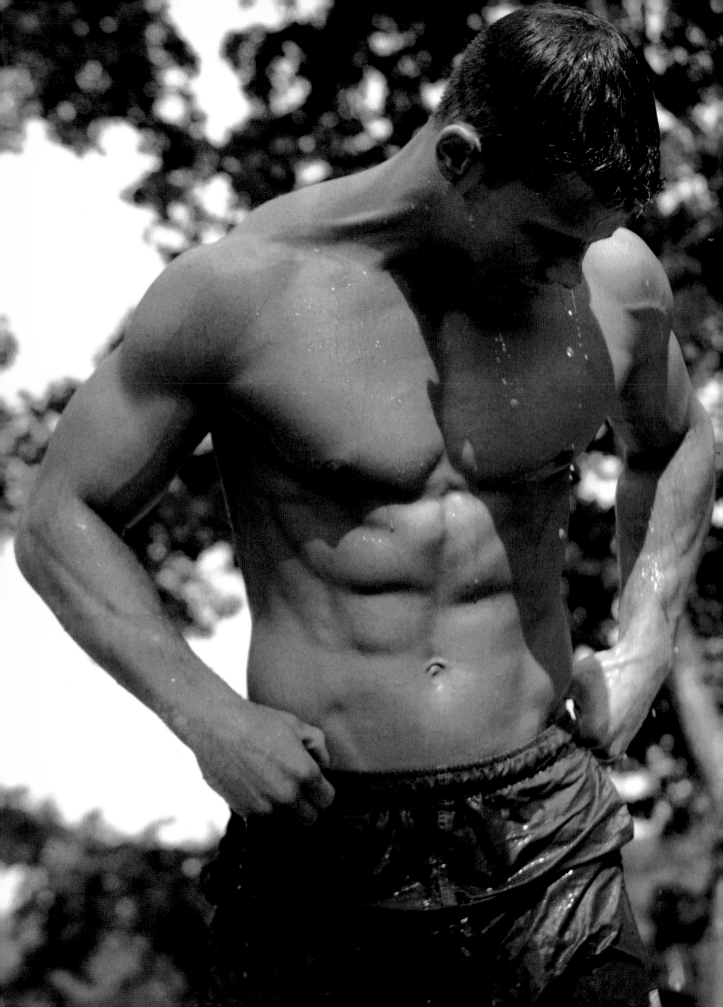

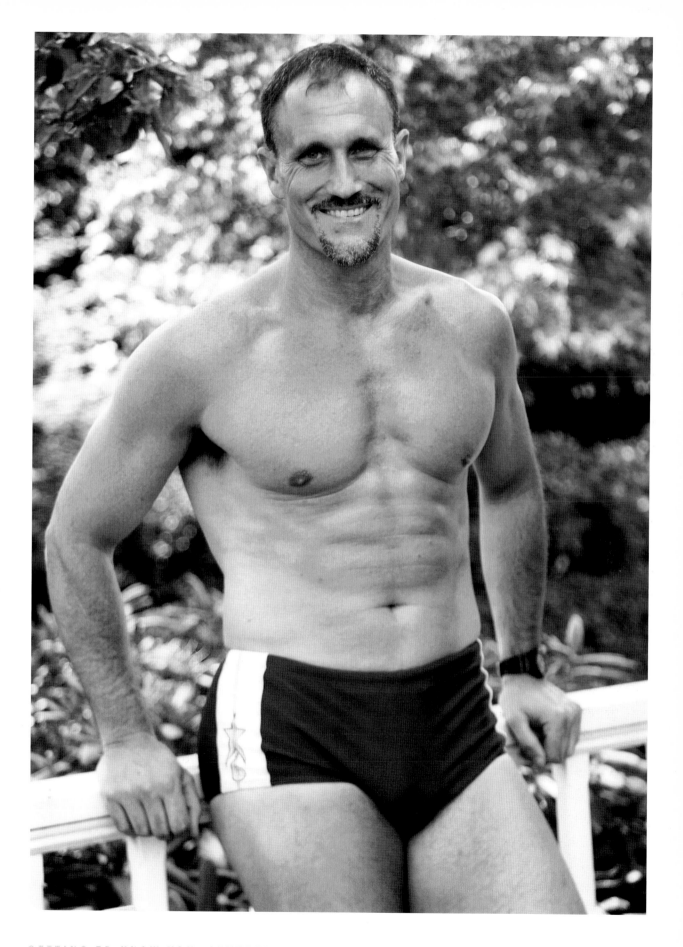

Take your pulse periodically during an exercise session to gauge your intensity level. Typically, the easiest location for taking a pulse is on the side of your neck, the carotid pulse. Be sure not to press too hard on the carotid artery or you'll get an inaccurate reading. Count the number of beats, always beginning with zero, for six seconds (then multiply by ten), or for ten seconds (then multiply by six) to get the number of times your heart is beating per minute. If your pulse is within your training heart-rate zone, you're right on track! If not, adjust your exercise workload until you get into your zone.

RATING PERCEIVED EXERTION (BORG SCALE)

Another method that can be used in conjunction with taking your pulse is Rating Perceived Exertion (RPE). This is a subjective method that allows you to determine how hard you feel you're working. RPE can be the primary means of measuring exercise intensity if you do not have typical heart-rate responses to graded exercise. Some exercisers may only be able to use the Borg Scale. These people include those on beta-blocking medications, some cardiac and diabetic patients, pregnant women, and others who may have an altered heart-rate response.

On a scale of 0–10, rate how you're feeling in terms of exercise fatigue, including how you feel both physically and mentally. You should be exercising between an RPE of 4 (somewhat strong) and an RPE of 5 or 6 (strong). Use the following table to determine the intensity level:

0	NOTHING AT ALL
0.5	VERY, VERY WEAK
1	VERY WEAK
2	WEAK
3	MODERATE
4	SOMEWHAT STRONG
5	STRONG
6	STRONGER
7	MUCH STRONGER
8	VERY STRONG
9	VERY, VERY, STRONG
10	STRONGEST

THE TALK-TEST METHOD

Like the RPE, the talk-test method is subjective and should be used in conjunction with taking a pulse. The talk test is quite useful in determining your comfort zone of aerobic intensity, especially if you are just beginning an exercise program. If you are able to talk during your workout without having a labored breathing pattern, you're most likely in your comfort zone.

TIME—THE BEST TIME TO EXERCISE

Contrary to popular belief, women aren't the only ones with biological clocks. We all have them and heed their ticking on a daily basis. If you are a regular

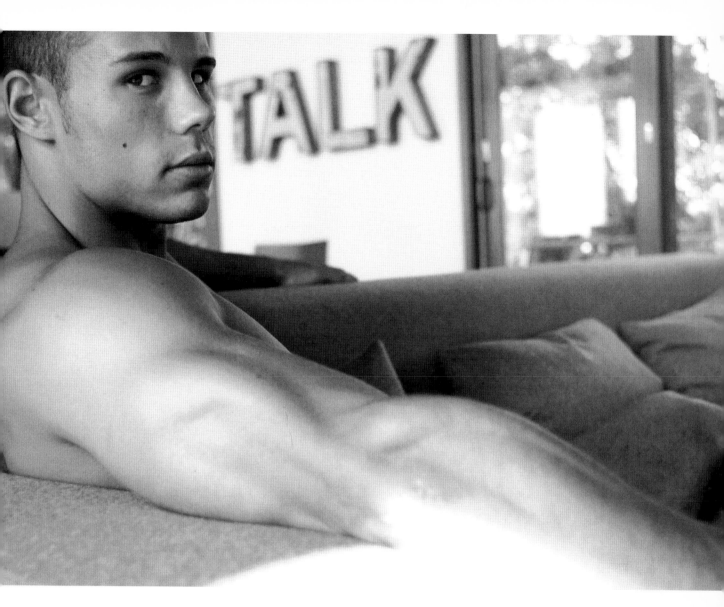

exerciser, you may already be aware of your most productive time to exercise and follow a routine that works best for you. On the other hand, if your exercise time varies from day to day, and it's wearing you out instead of pumping you up, you may be interested in studies of the proverbial internal clock and how to best determine what time of day you should schedule your workouts.

that our bodies follow. These rhythms originate in the hypothalamus and regulate everything from body temperature and metabolism to blood pressure. The rhythms result from the firing rate of neurons. They have conformed to our twenty-four-hour, light-to-dark cycle and may be regulated and reregulated each day according to the environment.

WARM IS BETTER

RHYTHM: IT'S NOT JUST FOR DANCING

The secret lies in circadian rhythms, the daily cycles

The influence of circadian rhythms on body temperature seems to yield the most control over the quality of a workout. When body temperature is at its highest, your workouts will likely be more productive; when body temperature is low, your exercise session may be less than optimal. Body temperature is at its lowest about one to three hours before most of us wake up in the morning. In the late afternoon, body temperature reaches its peak. Studies have consistently shown that exercise during these late-in-the-day hours produces better performance and more power. Muscles are warm and more flexible, perceived exertion is low, reaction time is quicker, strength is at its peak, and resting heart rate and blood pressure are low.

DON'T FIX IT IF IT'S NOT BROKEN

Don't change your schedule if you feel good beginning your day with exercise. Everyone agrees that exercise at any time is better than no exercise at all. In fact, people who exercise in the morning are more successful at making a habit of it. And though it has been suggested that morning exercise may put some people at higher risk for heart attacks, further research indicates that there is simply a generalized increased risk of heart attacks in the morning. If your schedule favors an early workout, emphasize stretching and a good warm-up to ensure that your body is ready for action.

OTHER CONSIDERATIONS

If stress relief is your goal, exercise always works, all the time. And if you're wondering when it's best to train for an upcoming event, it all depends on what time you'll actually be competing. If an upcoming marathon begins at 7:00 A.M., try training at that time of day. Though training at any time of day will raise performance levels, research has shown that the ability to maintain sustained exercise is adaptive to circadian rhythms. In other words, consistently training in the morning will allow you to sustain exercise during a morning marathon longer than if you train in the evening.

FIND YOUR PEAK

To determine your own circadian peak in body temperature, record your temperature every couple of hours for five to six consecutive days. Body temperature usually fluctuates by plus or minus 1.5 degrees throughout the day. Try exercising during the period three hours before and after your highest temperature. If you are an early bird or a night owl, you may notice that your temperature peaks one to two hours before or after the norm (between 4:00 P.M. and 6:00 P.M.); you can adjust your exercise time accordingly.

TOO MUCH OF A GOOD THING

A little exercise is good for you, so more must be better, right? Well, sometimes. And sometimes more is just that—more. There comes a point of diminishing returns, or worse, a point where your body says *enough!*

Every one reaches this point at different times. Triathletes, for example, are able to withstand the rigors of three-sport training—running, cycling, and swimming—at levels unthinkable to most. For others, an extra step class or hitting the weights too hard can put them over the top. In the quest for better health and fitness, it is sometimes difficult to quell one's enthusiasm and take a break from exercise. But if exercise is leaving you more exhausted than energized, you could be suffering from a case of overtraining.

KNOW THE SIGNS

It's important to be able to recognize the signs of overtraining before they become chronic. Physical signs of overtraining include:

- Decreased performance
- Loss of coordination
- Prolonged recovery
- Elevated morning heart rate
- Headaches
- Loss of appetite
- Muscle soreness/tenderness
- Gastrointestinal disturbances
- Decreased ability to ward off infection

Keep in mind that not all of the signs of overtraining are physical. Much as regular exercise has a positive effect on mood and stress levels, too much exercise can do just the opposite, leaving the exerciser irritable and depressed, particularly as the quality of the workouts declines. Psychological and emotional signs of overtraining include depression, apathy, difficulty concentrating, emotional sensitivity, and reduced self-esteem.

UNDERSTAND THE CAUSE

Once you recognize the symptoms of overtraining, it's important to understand and honestly confront the cause. For some, overtraining occurs as a result of an upcoming competition. Increased training prior to an event is understandable, but if it's interfering with your health and well-being, you have to question its worth. The solution may be as easy as reducing the rate at which you increase your training intensity. The body needs sufficient time to adjust to your increased demands. Triathletes don't start out running ten miles, cycling one hundred miles, and swimming more than half a mile all at once. They gradually increase their training to allow their bodies to adapt.

For others, the basis for overtraining may have more to do with emotional or psychological reasons than physical ones. Exercise addiction is now recognized as a legitimate problem. Exercising beyond the point of exhaustion, while injured, or to the exclusion of all other aspects of one's life—these are some of the signs of exercise addiction. It's a difficult problem to recognize, particularly in a culture where discipline and control are lauded.

Individuals who exercise excessively are risking more than poor performance: They're risking their health. Overuse syndrome, which may lead to more serious injuries, is common. And the emotional cost of isolating oneself in order to exercise can be devastating. If you recognize these symptoms in yourself or in a friend, it is essential that you seek professional help.

THE M WORD—MODERATION

The key, it seems, to staying healthy is to do everything in *moderation,* which is best viewed as exercise relative to one's own fitness level and goals. Don't expect to exercise an hour every day simply because your very fit friend does. The body needs time to adjust, adapt, and, yes, even recuperate. Exercising to the point of overtraining is simply taking one step forward, two steps back—not exactly good training tactics.

Numerous people have asked me how I stay motivated to work out on a regular basis. After I list all the traditional motivational tips, which should be enough to make us all pull on our work-out clothes and work up a good sweat, I'm compelled to add my last resort—*pure determination!* I'm not unlike anyone else. There are days when I need to work out, but I simply can't muster the motivation to get my rear in gear. At those times, I look inward and draw from my pure determination to get myself moving.

I'm convinced that determination is what separates fitness as a "lifestyle" from fitness as a "hobby." If I view working out or weight training as a hobby, then I'm going to do it only when I *feel* like it. Defining something as a hobby implies an activity that you do in your spare time because you enjoy it. This definition doesn't completely work for me where fitness is concerned. Yes, I truly enjoy the benefits of fitness. However, I don't always truly enjoy the activity required to attain those benefits.

Viewing fitness as a lifestyle has completely changed my mental programming. Working out is an integral component of my life now. When something becomes part of your lifestyle, you do it whether you feel like it or not. It becomes a necessity. You know—like breathing!

I caution you not to program yourself to be obsessive either. Find the middle ground. Enjoying a few days off from working out is healthy. Your body needs rest. Working out four to five days per week is a good balance for me. You'll need to find your balance as well, and once you do, make it a part of your lifestyle. On those occasions when it's time to work out and you're completely devoid of motivation—look inward and draw from your *pure determination!*

HOW WE LEARN

People learn in different ways. Some people learn by watching someone else perform a task or job, some by listening to instructions. Others may need a hands-on approach. With this book, you will have the advantage of all three methods.

AUDIBLE = HEAR IT. There are people who can hear information and process it without ever looking at a photo, take direction well, and understand a verbal description after hearing or reading it once. The audible learner will learn the methods in this book through words. The text is conversational. I try to describe every exercise clearly so that there are no gray areas and so you will know when to breathe, where to feel your weight, and where you should feel the work.

VISUAL = SEE IT. The imagery in this book will provide you with a clear illustration of how each exercise will look. If you're a visual learner, you can look at something once and never hear a word describing the movement or placement. You'll get it when you see it.

KINESTHETIC = FEEL IT. The kinesthetic learner has to be touched. They respond in a way that needs more attention than I can provide via a book. A photo cannot reach out and touch you, and words may not be able to convey to your brain what the touch of a spotter or someone who can correct your form with their hands can do. I must trust that you will try your best at each of the exercises, and if you need help with any of the exercises, ask someone in your local gym for assistance.

CHAPTER THREE

JOURNALING: DEFINING MOMENT

Writing is a powerful tool. It helps us think, remember, and organize. It helps us focus in a way that thinking alone can't. Take a few moments to think about yesterday. Right now. Take a piece of paper and write about it: when you got up, what you did, the weather, who you saw, what you ate, the quality of the food, who you talked to and about what, what you thought about, and what made you smile or troubled you.

On another piece of paper write about tomorrow as if you had a crystal ball and could watch yourself going through the actions of the day. Look at tomorrow as a reflection of yesterday. What about tomorrow shows that you learned something about yesterday? Notice how much more you thought about what you recognize or visualize when you write it down. How powerful is that? Writing helps get beyond our mental barriers and exposes us to our true thoughts and memories.

A memorable visit from my eldest nephew helped me realize that a writing exercise can help us think out some of the clutter that alters our real experience. My nephew came to New York for a visit after fifteen years away. As he was leaving, I prompted him to write on his flight back to the Twin Cities. Instead of relying on the photos that he took to remind him of his experience, I gave him a journal so he could take the time on the plane to record his experience. I was delighted to find out that not only did he fill the journal, but he found a way to express only to himself his true feelings and desires. It was a vivid example of the power of writing. In this age of the computer and other electronic devices, of course you can record thoughts in a Palm Pilot or handheld device, but to nurture you with honest words and thoughts may require pen and paper.

Any attempt at well-being engages both mind and body. I encourage you to begin recording your thoughts and accomplishments in a journal. This is not a "dear diary" type of exercise, but a way for you to jot down the things that really matter and achievements that you make each day, as simple as some of them may be. There is no other record that is as true as one that records in our own words. Even photographs cannot tell us how we were feeling at the time they were taken.

Start by using a simple notebook or journal. Divide the first page into two columns. Title the left side of the column "HERE" and the right "THERE," or "TODAY" and "TOMORROW," or "PRESENT" and "FUTURE," or any other reference that works for you. This tool will help you define where you are now and what you want to achieve in the defined future. You have to

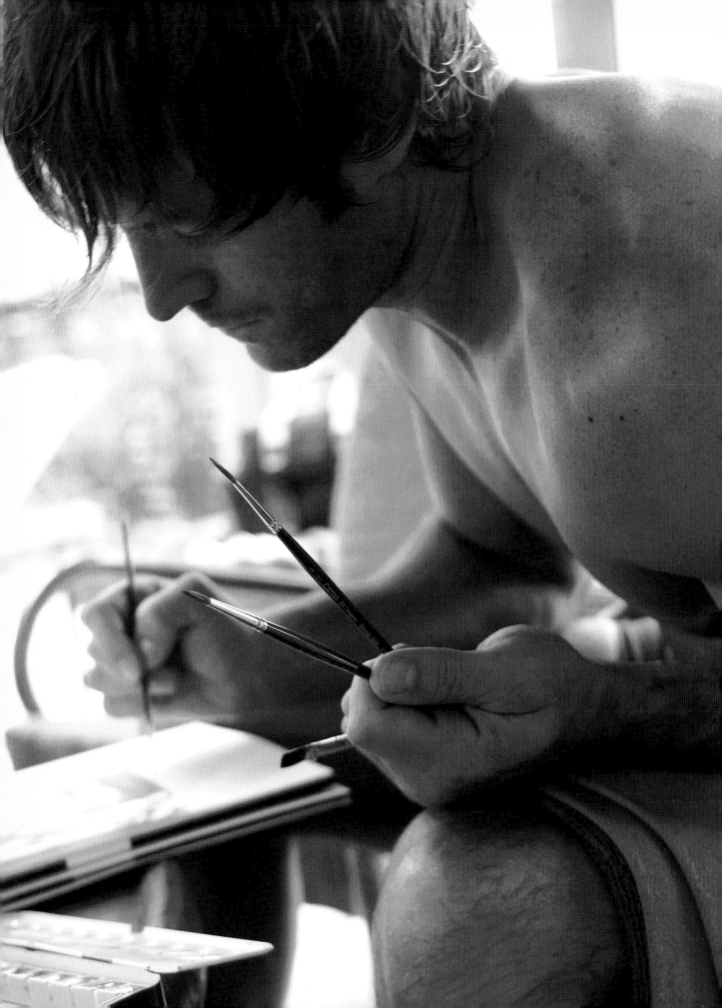

decide what you want before you can determine how to get it. With that in mind, in the left column write specific concerns you have. Try not to make general statements like, "I want to look better," or, "I want a better job"; but rather specific ones like, "I want to gain five pounds of muscle," or, "I want to find a job that allows me to travel more."

On the right side, list those steps you know are needed to accomplish the goal, list the activities or resources that will help accomplish the goal, and give yourself a reasonable time frame for successfully completing them. Finally, review your list carefully and prioritize each item in the left column. The first item is, for now, the only item to begin working on.

Start a new page in your journal (for now, write only on the right-hand pages, leaving the left pages blank). Title it with your first goal, and write yourself a contract. Writing a contract may seem a bit formal, but anything put in writing has a powerful effect. Think of the contract as a written promise you make to yourself.

Here is a sample:

I,_____, recognize the proven benefits of regular exercise and will from _____ (date) take the following steps to prepare myself to begin a fitness program:

1. I will walk one-half hour each day between the hours of _____ (time) and _____ (time).

2. I will increase my walking time by fifteen minutes each week to a maximum time of one hour.

3. I will discuss with _____ (friend or support person) the progress I have made each week as well as anything that has worked against my goal and why.

At the completion of each successful week, I will _____, (buy a CD, book, go to a movie, take in a baseball game). At the end of ninety consecutive days, I will _____ (*something big*: take a road trip or attend a concert).

Each day I do not complete my assigned task(s), I will deposit $2.00 into an envelope addressed to a charity or institution that I believe in. I will mail this envelope monthly.

Write in your journal about a variety of other things as well. Record activities related to your goals. Jot down your feelings, your actions, new ideas, discussions you have had with others. You don't have to be perfect here either. This is your personal book and can be used to write about anything you wish. A very important teacher told me, "A bad idea on paper is much better than a good idea in your head." You might be amazed at the results you find in your journal alone.

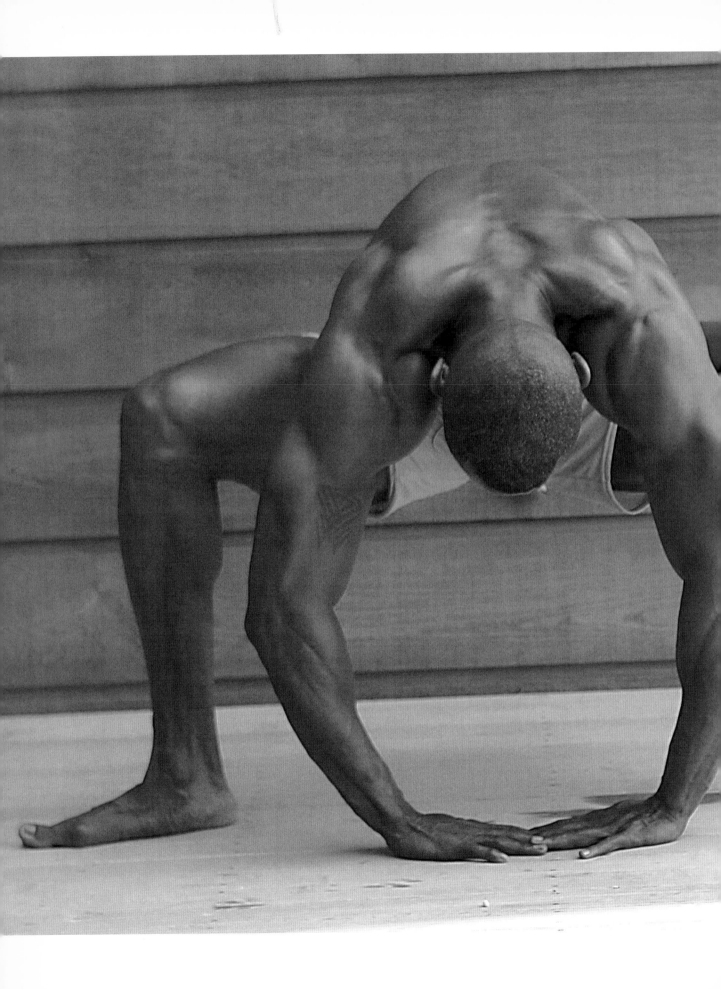

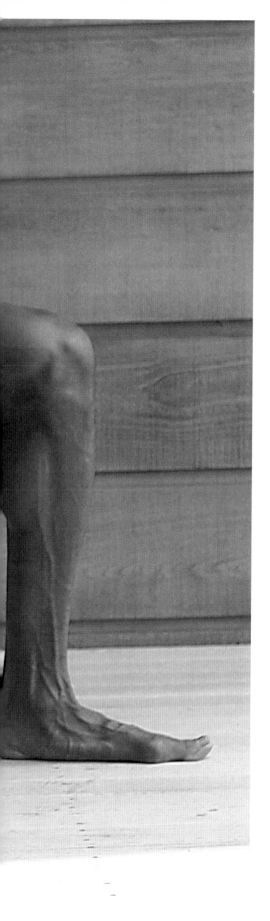

PART TWO

GETTING PHYSICAL:

PERFORMANCE

These rules to train by apply to all the strategies in this book.

POSTURE AND WEIGHT POSITIONS

POSTURE—CENTRAL POSITION. Central Position is a perfect postural position that should be maintained at all times. Ideal spinal alignment will offer numerous benefits not only for a fitness regimen but in many aspects of your life. Central Position is the foundation of safe and effective exercise technique.

Central Position involves equal contractions of the front and back of your legs in order to support the vital knee joints. It activates the buttocks and hips to support and maintain the pelvis' position and keeps your hips aligned. All of the muscles around your torso contract to support the middle spine to keep the spine in a neutral, natural position. Your chest supports the upper part of the spine, and your neck supports the head.

Position feet directly under your shoulders. Turn them out slightly. Keep your knees slightly bent and your butt tucked under you. Try not to exaggerate the tuck; it should feel comfortable. Hold your torso firm and support your chest high. Pull your shoulders back as if you were carrying an egg between your shoulder blades. Pull your head back just a little, allowing your chin to relax. In yoga Central Position is called "the Mountain"; in the armed forces, it is called "Attention."

A NEW WAY TO SIT

Everyone knows that Americans are becoming more sedentary. Innovations in everything from dishwashers to computers have made our lives easier. This decline in physical activity is having very negative effects on our health. Using a ball as a chair in your home or office is a simple, yet effective way to add some activity to your life, especially if you spend a lot of time at a computer!

Take a minute and, without moving, think about how you are sitting. Are you slumped back into a chair? Slumped sideways? How often are you in this position? Have you ever thought about what it might be doing to your back and your overall health?

Poor posture leads to uneven loading of disks in the spine and a compression of respiratory and digestive organs. Also, most chairs support your weight as you relax and, while this may be more comfortable, the support decreases the strength of the muscles that support your spine. This decrease in strength can lead to back pain or put you at risk for a back injury.

The stability ball promotes "active sitting" because you cannot relax while seated on it. There are constant small adjustments in your back, hips, knees, and ankles to keep you balanced. These small adjustments help circulation to the disks in your spine and can strengthen your back muscles. Also, gentle bouncing on the ball will encourage you to sit in the correct posture and will strengthen your postural muscles.

Foot placement can and will have a direct effect of how easy or difficult you want each exercise with the ball to feel. With your feet separated on the floor in front of you, each foot acts like a kickstand on a bike. The wider apart your feet are, the easier it is to sit on the ball. As you draw your feet inward, your torso must stabilize in order to stay on top of the ball.

By positioning your feet together in front of you,

any seated exercise will require you to use maximum muscle systems to stay on the ball. Each exercise that is either seated (upright), bridged (supine), or facing down (prone) will offer a variety of levels for you to utilize. Start with your feet separated about hips' distance for the first set of any exercise to establish your technique and then make advancements gradually and systematically simply by bringing your foot position closer together.

BRACE YOURSELF

I like to use this technique for everything from pressing a weight into the air to setting up an exercise, from supporting a stretch to taking off my shirt in public. I use the last example to appeal to your ego, so you can really "get it." What is the first thing you automatically do when you take off your shirt? You suck in your gut! Even if you don't have one, I'll wager you do this anyway. You pull in your abs as a guarantee that you are sporting a six-pack, a four-pack, or just putting your best belly forward. Channel this automatic response into training with a braced midsection.

In a standing position, place your thumbs on your lowest ribs and your middle fingers on your pelvic bone. Your hands will be placed palms against your side. Now inhale a full breath and exhale. You should feel your middle fingers and your thumbs pinch together when you exhale. Try it again and feel how your abs stretch and contract when you breathe. The end of the exhale or breathing out portion is *bracing yourself*. When you lift or position your body on the ball or the floor, even on a piece of weight-training equipment, I feel it is necessary to brace yourself for the upcoming exercise that requires you to support your spine and contain your body movement.

MOVING AWAY FROM THE CENTER

Intensity levels are adjustable on the stability ball by simply positioning the ball away from the center of your body. When you are sitting upright on the ball, your spine will align itself to accommodate your balance. When you walk forward and lie back on the ball with your lower back resting against it (the supine position), resting farther away from the center of your lower back will determine how hard your abdominal region must work. This holds true for the position of the ball up toward your shoulders or toward your buttocks. Try it.

If you turn over into the prone position, with your hands flat on the floor in a push-up position with the ball in the center of your body, the farther away from your navel or hip area the ball is the more intense every exercise becomes.

HOW TO LIFT

It may seem like the easiest thing in the world, but lifting something off the floor, as you will be lifting weights off the floor, requires a few simple reminders. Size up the load and decide if the weight is too heavy or inappropriate for you to lift alone. Keep the weight close to your feet so that the load won't cause undue stress to your lower back, as it would if you lifted the weight too far from your center of gravity. Bend at the knees using your arm strength and leg strength to lift the load off the floor, keeping your chest lifted and your back supported.

Your back can be as strong as a girder in a building or as sensitive as a twig. You should always consider the weight before you lift it. Once your back is injured, it is more apt to get injured again. The vertebrae and the disks are a perfectly built piece of architecture; don't mess around with them.

When sitting on the stability ball and lifting, always roll forward slightly to grab the weight you are using with the same focus on contracting the abdominals and buttocks to keep you in position. When you finish each set, release the weights to a position that will keep them available. You could also consider using a hand weight that has eight-edge weights on the ends to prevent them from rolling away.

WEIGHT: PLUS OR MINUS

Selecting the appropriate weight is often a problem with many programs. Don't take any suggestions without knowing that you have a choice. Select a weight that allows you to perform the right number of repetitions for the program you have decided on. For general good health and balance, The American College of Sports Medicine (ACSM) recommends that you perform three sets of twelve repetitions per muscle group.

Start by lifting a weight that you think will be right for you. If you can lift those weights only six times, and the fifth and sixth were heavy, try another lighter set. If you can throw those weights across the room, go for heavier ones. Test everything out before you buy it. Buy a barbell that you can load and unload. That way you will be able to add and take off weight for different routines.

Remember, the amount of weight and the number of reps determine what type of training goals you are working toward. It is a good idea to start with a general program for about eight to ten weeks. Your muscle systems and cardiorespiratory system will be conditioned and ready for a challenge after that, and you'll feel the progress. Then switch your program to either strength or endurance. The variety will be good for you and will offer you new adaptations in the weeks to come.

The number of sets also determines the gains you experience. Even one set of repetitions with the appropriate weight should produce gains for most men. Between three and five sets are recommended for maximal gains. That's why you're here, right? To get and see change. Give yourself about one minute of rest between sets. This will give your body enough recovery time before performing the next set. If you wait too long, your body will cool off and your heart will slow down. You want to remain in a training mode. Longer rest periods waste time and create a pointlessly longer work-out session. Make the most of your time, and then get out of there.

PROGRESS

Science tells us you must overload your muscles in order to develop strength. You have to force the muscle to contract near the maximum tension to produce the physiological modifications necessary for change to occur. Otherwise the muscle will not increase in size or strength, but will adapt only to the load it is subjected to. Max = maximum gains. Minimal = minimal gains. More effort on your part will produce more of you!

DUMBBELL POSITION (SIDE OF BODY). Hold each dumbbell with a relaxed grip. Try not to squeeze the metal to the point where it hurts just to hold the weight. Exercise gloves will give you a better grip, and I encourage you to wear them whenever you are lifting. As you drop down to pick up the dumbbells, squat down as you would if you were picking up a fragile package. You'll perform the task with greater attention to "the package" and your back. Bend both knees and keep your back supported until you grasp the weights, then lift with the legs. This helps avoid any undue stress to the lower back area. Then return to your Central Position.

Hold the dumbbells at your sides with your shoulders relaxed and your torso contracted to avoid the arching of your lower back. If the weights are too heavy, your body will also tell you when to put them down.

BARBELL POSITION—OPTIONAL. Barbells can be used in place of hand weights. Do not load the bar too heavily to start. The barbell will most always be sitting on the floor in front of you, so use the same technique that is described for the dumbbells. Bend at the knees with your shoulders up, never bend from the waist to pick up them—or anything else.

When holding the barbell on your shoulders behind the neck, it is important for you to be aware of a few tips that will promote the best technique for you to use to ensure safety and comfort. Bring the barbell onto the shoulders carefully and rest the weight of the barbell on the meaty part of your upper back, also known as the trapezoids or "traps." This position will help you to avoid resting the barbell on the vertebrae at the upper part of your back and lower part of your neck. You don't want to bruise that part of your body. If you need a cushion, wrap a towel around the barbell. Try to hold the barbell with relaxed hands positioned below the shoulders. This will assist your support of the barbell without causing you to tilt or bend forward when you perform exercises.

WHAT'S THE FREQUENCY?

Now that you have an idea of how many sets and reps to perform the question of how often arises. Because we are talking about something you have to do regularly, it can sound a little overwhelming. For a beginning weight-training program, the general rule is to lift weights three times per week. A schedule could be Monday, Wednesday, and Friday or Tuesday, Thursday, and Saturday. This gives you a day off between sessions for rest—and you'll need it. Your body deserves it! You want to concentrate on working each body part (legs, back, chest, shoulders, biceps, triceps, abdominals) with your desired exercises. That doesn't mean you do every exercise in this book three times a week. Take one exercise for each body part and hit it with three sets. This is the best way to set yourself up with a program and to get used to the whole idea of working out. Then move on to the next body part. It's simple.

A split routine means that you do just that. Split the work—but that doesn't mean you are doing half the work. In fact, it means the opposite. You perform multiple exercises (more than one) for specific body parts. You also double the number of sessions per week, but you alternate the work. For example, Monday, Wednesday, and Friday you might perform chest, back, and shoulder exercises. Tuesday, Thursday, and Saturday you would work legs and arms. This type of training is recommended for intermediate to advanced lifters.

To recap. For the beginning lifter, three times a week, one exercise per muscle group, three sets. When you become more advanced and conditioned, you can change your routine into a split routine, six sessions per week, with multiple exercises for specific muscle groups.

LET THERE BE ORDER

Exercise large muscle groups before you hit the smaller ones. Large muscle groups are legs (quadriceps, hamstrings), back, and chest. The smaller muscle groups assist the big boys. To begin a routine with biceps curls could possibly result in an injury and over stressing the arm. Also, the large muscle groups rely on the support of the smaller muscles, so if you exhaust them at the beginning of the session, you risk compromising the entire program.

Set up your exercises so that you don't continually recruit the same muscles to help assist in the next exercise. This offers a bit of rest to the group you just worked to fatigue.

ONE SIDE VERSUS THE OTHER

Opposing muscle groups—it sounds like two teams playing in the Super Bowl! It is a bit like that. The back is in competition with the chest. The hamstrings are in competition with the quads. If you strengthen one side of your body, you should offer the same work to the other side. Balanced training can create better balance and a great physique. You see it sometimes in men on the street—all shoulders and chest but bird legs. Or legs like tanks and skinny arms. Many men will work on the muscles they feel most insecure about and hope the rest will follow along.

The best approach is equal time, balance, and harmony. Body parts work together to perform daily "functional" movements, so why show a preference to only one side in workouts? The body works as a whole. The programs in *Beyond Basic Training* will focus equal time on opposing muscles:

Front of the body/Back of the body

Shoulders/Latissimus dorsi

Chest/Back

Biceps/Triceps

Quadriceps/Hamstrings

Abdominals/Lower back

ABOUT YOUR BREATH

We breathe about 900 times per hour, about 21,600 times per day, and about 7,844,000 times per year. It is the most fundamental function, but we rarely give it a second thought. Breathing can be a powerful tool. If we learn how to use it, it can literally change our physiology in very dramatic ways. Breathing is one of the few body functions that is under both our conscious and unconscious control. In other words, we can willfully deepen or hold our breath, or we can forget about breathing altogether and it will continue on, using the nervous system's equivalent of automatic pilot, the autonomic nervous system (ANS).

The ANS has two main branches that govern the unconscious functions of our bodies. The "rest and digest" (parasympathetic) branch is responsible for healing, digesting, eliminating waste, the immune system, and basic day-to-day functioning. The "fight-or-flight" (sympathetic) branch of the ANS is what kicks in when we perceive danger. If a vicious dog comes at you, the fight-or-flight response reacts. Your body prepares to protect itself; adrenaline surges through your body. This energy can be spent getting you out of immediate danger.

Many of us are stuck in the fight-or-flight mode and consequently live our lives as if we are being chased by that dog. Our health and peace of mind are seriously compromised as a result. Luckily, breathing allows us to manually shift our ANS back into the rest-and-digest mode.

Close your eyes for a moment and notice your breathing. Don't try to change it right away. Just become aware of what it is like. Is it shallow and short (in the chest area) or full and deep (lower into the stomach area)? Allow the breath to deepen. Start by pulling the breath deep into your belly, filling the lower part of the lungs. Gradually allow the breath to fill the belly and the middle of the chest. Finally, allow the breath to fill all the way up into the top of your lungs. Don't rush; allow the air to fill your lungs slowly. When you exhale, move just as slowly and allow your lungs to empty completely. Allow yourself to take ten full breaths and then open your eyes.

By taking time to breathe in this way each day, we can set the tone of our lives and keep our minds and bodies healthy and strong. We can also use this technique when we feel the stress of life bearing down and threatening to crush us. Breathing properly may not fix external problems, but it will certainly induce a state that is much more effective in dealing with a lot of what life throws our way.

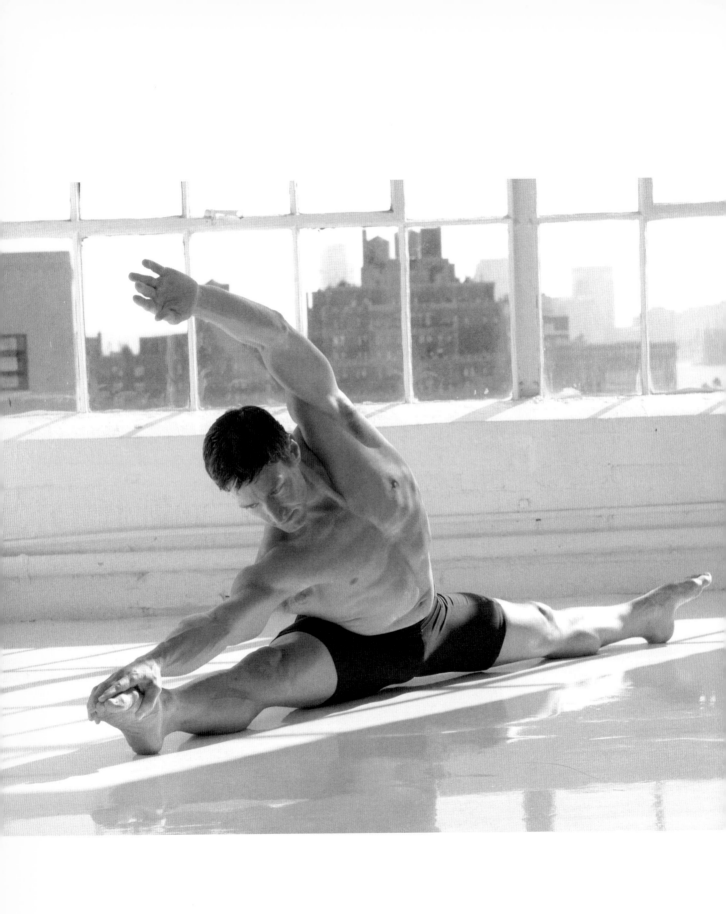

CHAPTER FOUR

PILATES-INSPIRED TRAINING

WHAT IS IT?

WHAT EXACTLY IS PILATES?

Joseph Pilates developed the Pilates method of body conditioning in Germany more than seventy years ago. For many years, Pilates training remained a well-kept secret in the world of dance and the performing arts. In recent years, the growing interest in "mind/body" exercise has brought Pilates's concepts to the forefront of fitness training. This wave of interest has seen stars such as Madonna, Sting, and Jodie Foster using the method and enjoying the benefits of Pilates training techniques.

The Pilates method comprises more than five hundred exercises, performed either as a mat-based workout or using special resistance equipment developed by Joseph Pilates and emphasizing spring resistance. The central concept of Pilates training is strengthening the so-called "powerhouse," or core, of the body—the deep abdominal muscles, buttock muscles, and the muscles around the spine. A training program based on Pilates will stabilize the pelvis and shoulder girdle, stretching and strengthening the entire body with movement initiating from "the center."

WHO WAS PILATES?

Joseph Hubertus Pilates was born near Düsseldorf, Germany, in 1880. As a child, he suffered from a number of physical ailments including rickets, asthma, and rheumatic fever. Pilates determined to overcome these health problems and so began a lifetime's dedication to physical fitness.

The original Pilates studio was founded in New York in the 1920s. Beginning with gymnastics, body building, and skiing, he also studied Eastern methods of training such as yoga and Zen meditation. As a teenager, he was in good enough physical condition to pose for anatomical charts—quite a transformation!

As, Joseph Pilates wrote: "We should recognize the mental functions of the mind and the physical limitations of the body so that complete coordination between them may be achieved." Pilates left his native Germany for England in 1912, where he earned a living in various ways: as a professional boxer, circus performer, even a teacher of self-defense to members of the police force at Scotland Yard. He continued to develop his system of exercise while interned during World War I. The origins of the modern-day "Reformer"—the most commonly used machine for Pilates, which resembles a bed with pulleys with its spring resistance and sliding carriage—are to be found in equipment that Joseph Pilates developed during the war to enable bedridden patients to continue to exercise and develop strength and flexibility, working with springs taken from their beds.

From the beginning, his greatest fans were drawn from the world of the performing arts. Leading lights of the dance world such as Martha Graham, George Balanchine, and Hanya Holm used the method to improve performance and prevent injury. Pilates continued to teach and develop equipment and exercises with his beloved wife, Clara, until his death in 1967. He was fond of speculating that in his theories and ideas he was fifty years ahead of his time. Given the universal popularity of Pilates training across the world at the start of the new millennium, he seems to have been right!

WHAT DOES "MIND/BODY" ACTUALLY MEAN?

Pilates formulated six basic principles for his exercise technique:

1. Breathing. The pattern of breathing is connected with the pattern of movement. It ensures a free flow of cleansing oxygen throughout the body, improves circulation, and helps to avoid unnecessary tension in the muscles.

2. Precision. The method emphasizes quality of movement over quantity.

3. Centering. Refers to the practice of initiating and controlling movement from the center or "Powerhouse"—abs, buttocks, and back muscles. This concept lies at the heart of Pilates's work.

4. Flowing movement. In combination with deep and relaxed breathing, the flowing movements in Pilates reduce stress on the body and the risk of injury.

5. Control. Vital! Momentum has no place in this method of training.

6. Concentration. In Pilates, the mind and the body work as a team. Every exercise requires your full attention. Observe your body as it works; think about each stage of movement.

WHAT IS SO SPECIAL ABOUT THE PILATES METHOD?

Traditional methods of training and developing the body tend to produce short, bulky muscles—precisely the type of musculature most prone to injury. Pilates elongates the spine, increasing the elasticity of muscles and the flexibility of joints. This balance between strength and flexibility drastically reduces the potential for injury. The method emphasizes flowing movements requiring the use of multiple muscle groups simultaneously. Controlled breathing and concentration are essential, making Pilates truly a workout for the body *and* the mind. It avoids the tendency of many exercise forms to emphasize the muscles that are stronger and neglect those that are already weaker. In this way Pilates can help your body to regain efficient patterns of motion—a great benefit to those recovering from injury, to professional athletes and performers, or to anyone seeking good posture and optimal health.

THE PURPOSE OF PILATES

Pilates creates its long, lean appearance because it strengthens and tones muscles without adding bulk. But aesthetics are minor compared to its other advantages.

Pilates makes you think. You have to become really acquainted with your body to practice Pilates properly. For example, you can repeatedly perform the

same move; but if you don't concentrate on holding your core stable, you won't experience the full
benefits of the practice.

BREATHING PREP. In a seated position on the floor, hold your legs
in toward your body with your
knees bent, your arms wrapped
around your thighs and your hands
down around your feet. Do not
hold too tight, as this is just a way
for you to take notice of each
breath you breathe. This should
also give you a chance to unwind
your entire back, lengthening your
spine and loosening your neck
muscles. Notice how each breath
fills your lungs. As you breathe out,
you will feel your abdominal region tighten. The goal here is to
draw air in and to push air out of
your lungs with intent and technique. This preparation is meant
for the practice and also as a way
for you focus on the session ahead.
Take in ten full breaths and then
begin your routine.

SPINAL ROLL UP. Lie in a supine
position face up on the floor. Feel
the full length of your body extending with your arms reaching to
one side of the room as your legs
extend to the other side. Breathe in
as you raise your arms to the ceiling
and begin the roll up. You have to

Spinal Roll Up 1

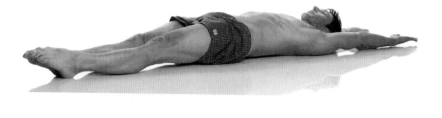

Spinal Roll Up 2

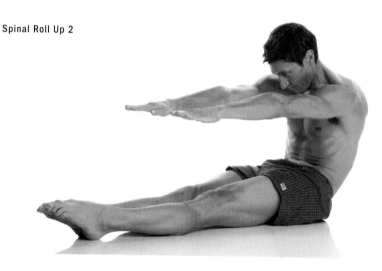

Spinal Roll Up 3

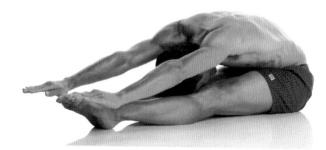

draw your chin down toward your
chest as you lift and continue to roll
your shoulders off the floor as you
breathe out. The difficulty is that

you must maintain the extension of
the legs while rolling up. If this creates uncomfortable stress in your
lower back, you can bend at the

knees. You should feel as though each vertebra is lifting individually like a link system. Lift all the way up to a full seat and then forward as far you can reach.

There are two benefits to the roll up. It will stretch your back at the same time it strengthens your entire abdominal region. Breathing here is also vital. Breathe out as you roll up, breathe in on the stretch forward, and breathe out on the roll back down. Perform ten roll ups in continuous repetitions. This will minimize the flexion of the psoas, a muscle that lies in front of the hip.

THE HUNDRED. Lie in a supine position face up on the floor. Feel the full length of your body extending with your arms reaching to one side of the room as your legs extend to the other side. Breathe in as you

The Hundred 1

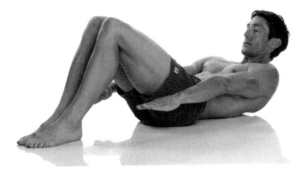

The Hundred 2

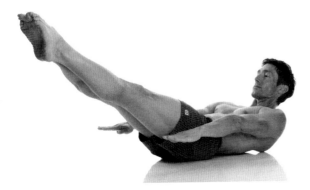

raise your head and shoulders to the ceiling and bend your knees, sliding your toes on the floor as they move. Bring your legs into the air on a diagonal while extending your arms past your hips with your palms facing down. Touch your legs together at the knees as you extend the hamstrings. Hold this position. Pinch your buttocks together slightly as you hold the position. Breathe in for five seconds, and breathe out for five seconds. Repeat ten breaths in and out without resting. Strength will become greater with practice. When you are able to perform the breathing rhythm up to ten-second breath in and ten-second breath out in two-set intervals, you will properly perform the Hundred.

Percussion breathing is what you see people doing when they are bobbing their arms down and up. This pumping assists the breathing count. Maintain the smooth breathing rhythm for five seconds. Each breath should be drawn in five counts exhaled out in counts while you press your hands down one hundred times equalling ten breaths.

DOUBLE LEG STRETCH. Lie on your back with your knees comfortably bent and pulled in to the chest. Hold your hands on your shins and elevate your head off the ground so that your eyes look at your knees. Your feet will be positioned near your buttocks. If you need additional support for your head, you can use a pillow or towel. Breathe in and prepare for the extension. As you breathe out, extend your arms forward through your hands, held about a half foot off the floor. On the same breath, extend both legs into the air at about a 45-degree angle. If you need to modify the position to ease lower back stress, keep your feet higher in the air. To challenge the abdominals or to intensify them, extend your legs closer to the floor. Try to maintain a flat back against the floor and pull your

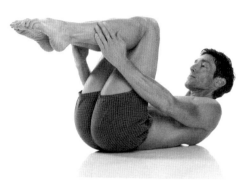

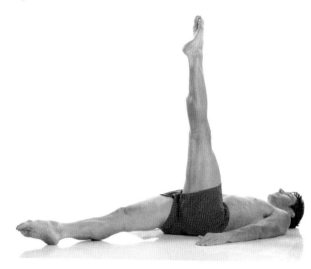

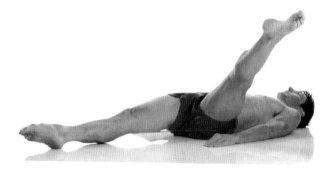

abs in (scoop them out). Take a breath as you lift your arms up into the air to reach a vertical position with your arms pointing up. Hold this for one second and breathe out as you pull your arms toward the back of the room. Hold this position for one second. Pull your ribs in again to ensure proper form. Return to the starting position on the floor while breathing in. Rest for only a moment before you start another repetition. Perform only in sets of ten reps.

LEG CIRCLES. Lie on the floor with both knees bent and your feet resting on the floor. Place your hands on the floor with your palms facing down and your elbows slightly bent. Stabilize your center by pulling

downward toward the floor with your ribs and feeling your spine print a pattern on the floor beneath you. Raise your right leg into the air with a pointed foot, which will contract the calf, and extend your leg just a bit farther than without the point. Press your other butt cheek into the floor. You will start by making counterclockwise circles with your leg. Think of it as drawing a circle on the ceiling with a pen that is sticking out of your toe. Breathing out as your leg crosses your body toward the left, you will feel your abs contract to assist the leg movement. Keep your leg extended and lower it to the floor, now stretching the abs. Swing your leg out to the far right close to the floor, and then bring your leg back into the position

Spinal Twist 1

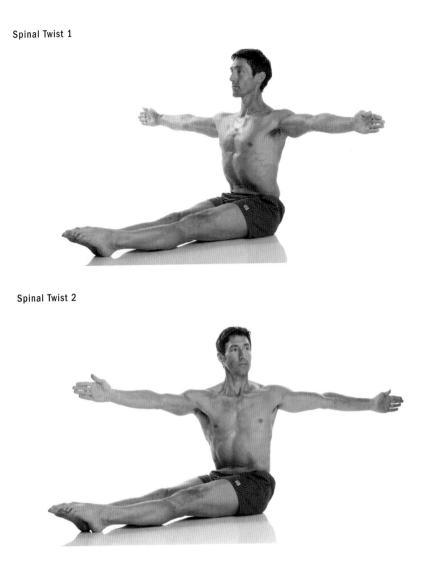

Spinal Twist 2

you started in. Try to prevent pushing your arms against the floor as this will create stress in your neck and shoulders and compromise your form. Try doing six circles per leg and then repeat the exercise in the other direction for both legs. You can also advance the exercise by extending your bent leg while drawing the circles with your active leg. Try this only after you have thoroughly practiced the basic exercise.

SPINAL TWIST. Sit up on your coccyx with tall posture, keeping your legs extended in front of you. Press through the toes of your feet and position them together. Lift your arms up to shoulder height without pulling your shoulders into the air. Keep your shoulders pressed downward as you extend your arms fully with your palms facing the front. Take a full breath in to prepare for the twist. Rotate your up-

per body as far to the right as you can, and pull your ribs down to maintain a tall posture. Imagine that your upper body is the handle of a key with your lower body inserted into a keyhole and try to keep the rotation only from the hips. After you rotate to one side, hold for one second and breathe out a little more, rotating just a bit farther, pulling your right shoulder blade back as far as possible. Breathe in as

Teaser 1

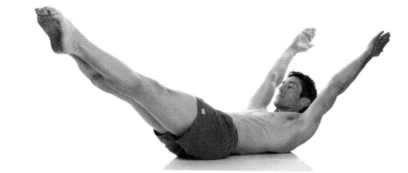

Teaser 2

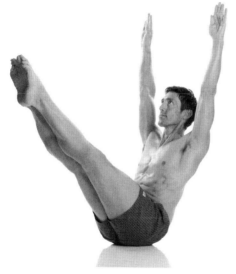

you return to the beginning position and, without hesitation, start rotating to the other side using the same technique. Turn your head with your shoulders to help the rotation. Start slowly as you learn this exercise, performing about ten rotations.

TEASER. Start this exercise in a seated position with your legs extended and your feet pointed out in front of you. Always maintain a slight pull of the knee caps to ensure your legs' position. Your arms should be at shoulder level, also extended in front of you. Breathe in and, as you do, lean your upper body back, rocking slightly to the back as you raise your legs into a V-shaped sit up. Lift your legs up to your head level or as close as you can get while you balance on your coccyx. Maintain a long neck and strong back for this difficult exercise. Pause for a second and then lower your legs back to the starting position. Repeat for eight to ten repetitions. Breathe out as you tilt back and in as you lower back down. The Teaser as illustrated here is advanced. You will start in a supine position, fully extended on the floor. Breathe in and, as you exhale, lift your legs and your arms simultaneously.

SIDE-LYING SIDE LEG LIFT. Start by lying down on your left side with your head resting in your hands or on your arms as if you were sleeping. Your body should be fully extended on the floor as if you were standing horizontally. This should provide you with a space between the floor and your waist. You will immediately feel a tightening when you engage this strict form for any side-lying exercise. You can rest your right hand on the floor in front of you at waist level. Tighten your buttocks to provide additional support of your lower back, and keep your toes pointed. Breathe out as you start the exercise by elevating your right leg (top leg) only. Hold your leg in the air for one second and then lower the leg as you breathe in, taking your leg back down to its starting position. Without complete rest, repeat. You will feel the pull of your thigh as well as the pull from your waist. The first stage of the exercise will help you to develop the movement skill, then advance by lifting both legs at the same time.

Side-Lying Side Leg Lift 1

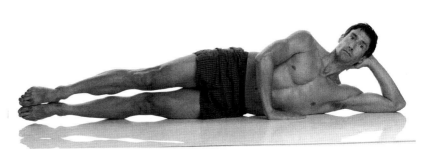

Side-Lying Side Leg Lift 2

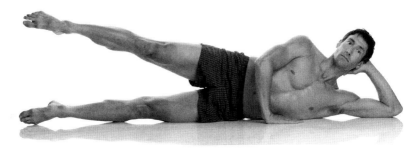

Side-Lying Side Leg Lift 3

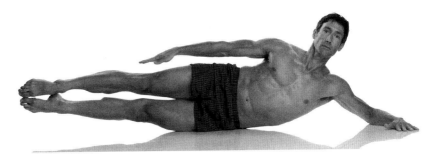

Hip Lift with Twist 1

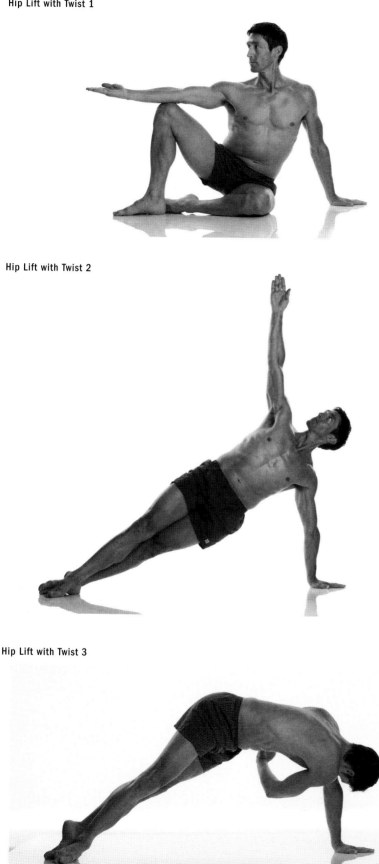

Hip Lift with Twist 2

Hip Lift with Twist 3

HIP LIFT WITH TWIST. Start by sitting on one side, keeping your legs bent, one knee on the floor and one in the air. Think of sitting at the beach and looking out to sea. Support yourself with one arm, your hand on the floor and the other arm resting on your knee. Lift through the hips, keeping your feet together. As you lift your hips into the air, raise your free arm up to the ceiling, directly above your shoulder. Your position will be similar to a side-lying "T" shape. Hold your body on the one hand with your torso tightly pulling all your muscles to support the position. Take a full breath in to prepare for the twist. Rotate your upper body as you reach down and under with your free arm to the area behind you. You will feel unsteady at first. Imagine a coil wrapping tight and then releasing in a spring action. Open your arm back up to the ceiling and return to the side-lying "T" position, maintaining a long spine and tight midsection. You should breathe in as you rotate to help facilitate the contraction of the lungs and the tightening of the abs. Start slowly with five lifts or so. If it's too much, you can do the same exercise on your knees maintaining the same position with your upper body and follow as described above. As you

Leg Pull 1

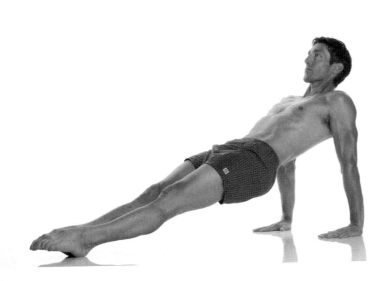

Leg Pull 2

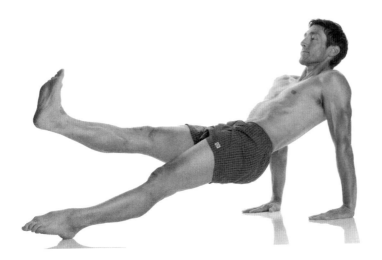

Saw

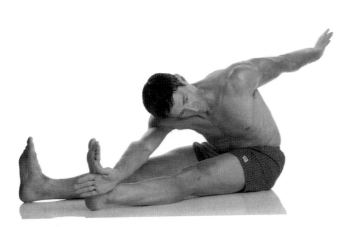

grow more proficient, build up to performing this exercise about ten times on each side.

LEG PULL. Sit up on your coccyx with tall posture, keeping your legs extended in front of you and your hands at your side on the floor, fingers pointing forward. With your feet positioned together and pointed, press through the heels of your hands and lift your torso into the air. Your body will become rigid, like a pier or a plank. The support should be directed from the shoulders, triceps, torso, and the buttocks. These are the muscles you need to support the middle of your body in this position. Keep your eyes focused directly forward. Lift one leg up into the air with a long and fluid movement. Think of it as pulling through water, smooth and consistent. As you bring your foot back down to the floor, flex your toes toward your body. Repeat the movement on one leg only ten to twelve times. Perform the same exercise on the other leg using the same direction as above.

SAW. Sit up on your coccyx with a tall posture, keeping your legs extended out in a 45-degree angle at your side. Press through the heels of your feet, and keep your knee caps pulled back to help you maintain the extension. Lift your arms up to shoulder height without pulling your shoulders into the air. Breathe in. Keep your shoulders pressed downward as you extend your arms fully with your palms facing the floor. Breathe out as you rotate your upper body as far to the right as you can and pull your ribs down to maintain a tall posture, at the same time, reaching with your left hand toward the outside of your right foot. Once you get into position, continue to breathe two short, sharp breaths and saw at your foot two times, which will help you stretch farther. Breathe in as you return to the upper position and set up for the next Saw on the other side. Do ten repetitions to a set, alternating as you perform them. Modify this if you need to by mimicking the sawing move over your foot until you become flexible enough to touch your ankle.

ABOUT THE CORE

The *core* is a set of deep postural muscles that assist the bones and ligaments to hold our bodies up against gravity. These muscles—the transversus abdominus (TA), multifidus, pelvic floor, and the diaphragm—form a cylinder or tin can around your torso. When recruited properly, they function as a unit and can be referred to as the "inner unit." The pelvic floor is the foundation, just like the foundation of a house. If it is overstretched or gripping and cannot relax or contract, we lack a solid base of support and cannot respond to changing loads. Without a solid base of support, we can easily lose our balance.

The *diaphragm* is the roof. With proper breathing techniques, we get more efficient oxygen exchange in our lungs and a better connection to the core.

The *transversus abdominus* and *multifidus* strap around the cylinder. They form a corset that wraps around the torso. The *transverses abdominus* runs from the lower six ribs and across the front of the pelvis. The *multifidus* is a deep, multisegmental muscle that courses the entire length of the spine from the coccyx to the neck. These two muscles should cocontract and work as a unit to tighten the midsection and give the spine a gentle lift, acting just as Scarlett O'Hara's corset did.

When the core, or inner unit, is not functioning, we start to use other muscles to help hold body alignment and posture. An example may be the internal/external obliques or gluteal muscles. This changes the body alignment, which increases the wear and tear on joints and exhausts muscles that are designed to move the body rather than hold the body.

HOW TO BRING CORE WORK INTO YOUR ROUTINE. Attend a workshop or hire a personal trainer who can teach you how to identify an aligned or neutral spine in lying, sitting, and standing positions. The next step is learning proper breathing techniques, how to isolate a contraction of each of the core muscles, and then draw on them as a unit. Then introduce your newfound knowledge to your regular fitness routine. At first, the intensity and duration of this routine will decrease, but in a short period of time you will be stronger and more powerful than ever.

THE TRUTH ABOUT ABS

A slender midsection is not only desirable for aesthetic reasons, but also for health, lower-back protection, and to improve physical performance in sports. Which muscles should be exercised to trim the waist? Are the "six-pack" muscles of the abdomen the key to a flat stomach? How can we train in the most efficient and enjoyable way? The answers may surprise you.

Does exercising the abdominal "six-pack" help reduce waist size?

When we think of a trim midsection, strong abdominal muscles (in scientific terms, the *rectus abdominis*) naturally come to mind. Let's check this proposition. Lie down on the floor with your calves elevated on a chair and put your hands on your stomach. In this position, your stomach should be very flat. Yet your abdominals seem relaxed and even stretched. Now, contract your abs by lifting your shoulders from the floor without moving your lower back. As your abs flex, your formerly flat stomach tends to protrude. In other words, your abs tend to push your stomach out rather than in.

Now, position yourself on your hands and knees. Pull your stomach in as much as possible. You will feel that your abs are not involved in this maneuver. Conclusion: The abs have little to do with the size of your waist. Other muscles must be responsible. This is an opportunity, as these oft-neglected muscles (transversus abdominis, internal and external oblique), are easier to strengthen than the abs. Training them can quickly pull inches off your waist without dieting, while enhancing your physical capabilities and health.

IMPROVE PERFORMANCE AND PROTECT YOUR BACK

Three sets of muscles work in concert to flatten your stomach. They are: the *transverse abdominis* and the *internal* and *external obliques*. The first two muscles are not visible. All three are located to the right and to the left side of your *rectus abdominis* (ab muscles). They are covered by less fat, so it is easier to make them visible. As they become stronger, they will flatten your stomach. Both areas will give the impression that you carry a lean and thin midsection. These three muscle groups do not only possess aesthetic properties, they provide a very strong protection for the lower back. They are also involved in lateral flexion and body rotation. This last function is very important for physiological reasons. In everyday life, we often rotate our torso. This maneuver is a frequent cause of back injuries whenever the rotating muscles are underdeveloped and weak. In many sports, such as football, running, baseball, basketball, and so on, rotational power can make the difference between an average and a good athlete. Rotational exercises are often neglected, explaining poor performances and the high incidence of back injuries.

CLASSIC EXERCISES FOR THE STOMACH

BODY ROTATION This can be trained in two different ways! Either the torso rotates while the legs are fixed, or the legs rotate while the torso is fixed. The first classic exercise consists of a trunk twist: Lie on the floor, your hands behind your head with your legs bent at your knees, feet on the floor. Bring your right elbow toward the left knee. Lower yourself and repeat by bringing the left elbow toward the right knee. Repeat the movement.

REVERSE TRUNK TWIST. Lie on your back with your arms straight to your sides. Your legs should be up, straight, and forming a right angle with your torso. Slowly lower your legs to the right while keeping the leg/torso angle constant. Once you have reached the floor, use your rotational power to return to your starting position. Repeat by lowering your legs to the left. If you find this exercise too hard to perform, bend your knees slightly.

IMPROVED EXERCISES FOR A FLAT, FUNCTIONAL, AND STRONG STOMACH

EXERCISE BALL. The next chapter will provide more exercises. It is possible to solve all these problems and to greatly improve the effectiveness of rotational exercises with the help of an exercise ball. By lying on a ball (45–65cm) with your feet on the floor, the trunk twist takes on new meaning. The exercise ball should be placed under your lower back. Your feet should be spread apart on the floor. In this position, place your arms straight in front of your eyes. Twist your torso and your arms to the right and toward the rear in order to get maximal stretch. This stretching is very important to improve your flexibility and more closely duplicate the range of rotation needed in sports and to trigger a stretch reflex that will force more muscle fibers to contract.

Using your rotational strength, rotate to the left and forward. Try to go up as far as possible. Keep your eyes on your hands during the whole exercise. Don't bounce or jerk—movement should be smooth and slow. The greater range of motion allowed by the exercise ball will make this exercise much more productive. Compared to floor exercise, a workout on the exercise ball will permit you to go much farther forward and downward for greater stimulating effects. You can increase difficulty by rotating your legs in the opposite direction to that of your arms during the stretching phase. For even greater resistance, try holding an elastic band attached to a low, fixed point behind you.

The reverse trunk twist can also be significantly improved with the help of a the exercise ball. Place your torso on the ball while your hands hold two fixed points out to the side on the floor or behind you hold-ing a railing. Raise your legs at a right angle. Lower them to one side as much as your rotational strength allows. Return to the starting point and repeat. As your strength develops, your range of motion can be progressively increased for added stimulus. This exercise is safer than it looks because your hands take care of your balance. Once you are more comfortable with your stability, you can loosen your grip a little to create a more unstable environment. The ball makes this exercise fun and very comfortable. For added resistance, ankle weights can be added progressively.

You can either work both sides of your body simultaneously or work only one side at a time. If the latter, rest a little before training the other side. For purely aesthetic training, we suggest exercising one side at a time. For sports training, work both sides simultaneously. However, do not hesitate to alter your working pattern from time to time for variety.

Beginners should try two to three sets of trunk twists to gain muscle strength. As your rotational muscles strengthen, add one and then two sets of reverse trunk twists.

To strengthen for sports, three sets of each exercise should be performed at least twice a week. For aesthetic and back-protection training, three sessions a week are recommended. Once you can easily perform more than twenty repetitions, add resistance by increasing your range of motion by using elastic tubes or ankle weights. Don't rest more than one minute between sets.

As a starting rotational exercise for your training, alternate the reverse and the normal trunk twists. You can either perform all your sets as one exercise by itself or alternate one with the other after each set. Change your training pattern frequently for best results.

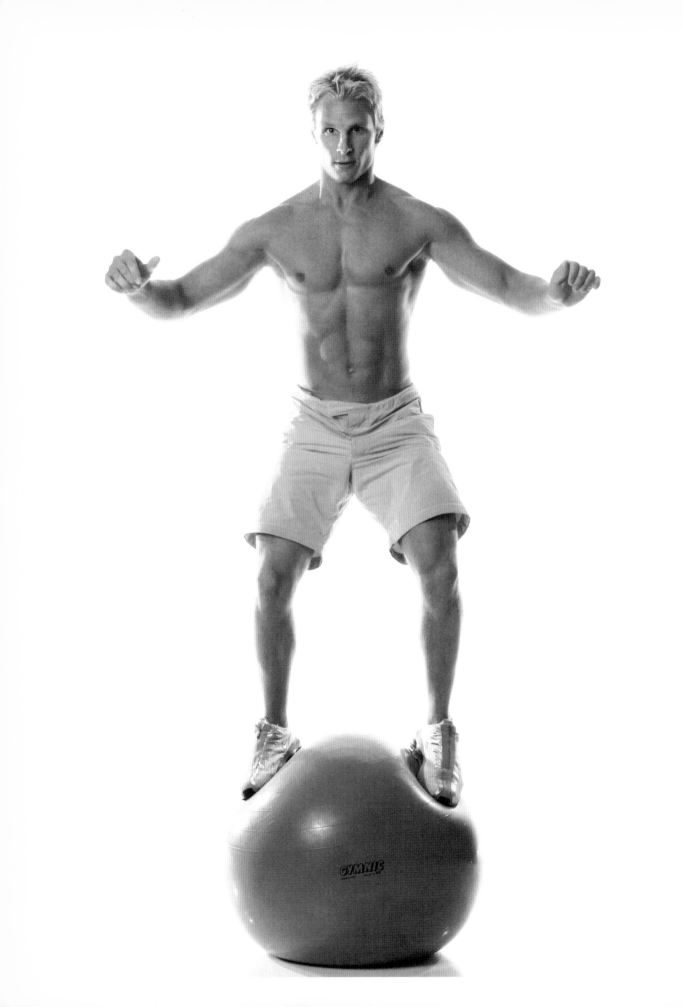

CHAPTER FIVE

STABILITY BALL TRAINING AND THE MEDICINE BALL

WHAT ARE STABILITY BALLS?

Big round exercise balls. Simple. Many people are reluctant to try exercise balls because they look and feel so unstable. They are . . . but that's the point. Training on a ball challenges your balance and is ideal for working your core muscles. When you do a chest press on a bench, you target isolated muscles in your chest and arms. But when you do that same exercise on a ball, you work your upper body and recruit stabilizing muscles—like the abdominals, glutes, and lower back—all at the same time. Apart from the fact that they can be a lot of fun, exercise balls help keep you motivated by adding variety to strengthening and stretching exercises. And since the ball helps build core strength, training with these inflatable orbs improves posture. Plus, ball training is easily adaptable to all levels of fitness.

If you can't get past your fear of falling off the ball (a natural first response), there are ways to ease into ball training. Softer or slightly deflated balls are less difficult to work with. Securing the ball against a wall or getting someone to hold it steady also helps alleviate anxiety. But remember, the more you secure the ball, the less stabilizing work your muscles have to do, which is the goal of using the ball in the first place.

HOW DO YOU CHOOSE THE RIGHT BALL?

SIZE MATTERS

Exercise balls come in a variety of sizes. Most fitness clubs carry 55-cm balls (the right size for most people between 5'0" and 5'7") and 65-cms balls (for most people between 5'8" and 6'2"). The best way to figure out the right ball for you is to sit on it. Your hips and knees should align at about a 90-degree angle.

Generally, the larger the ball, the easier it is to work with because there is more surface space as well as space between the ball and the floor. But size is important. Don't assume that all beginners should find the biggest exercise ball possible. Working with a ball that is too large may be easier for some exercises, but it makes others quite awkward and unsuccessful.

HOW YOU MEASURE UP . . . FOR THE RIGHT BALL (MEN AND WOMEN)

YOUR HEIGHT	BALL HEIGHT	BALL SIZE
Up to 4'10" (145 cm)	18 inches (45 cm)	Small
4'8" to 5'5" (140-65 cm)	22 inches (55 cm)	Medium
5'6" to 6'0" (165-85 cm)	26 inches (65 cm)	Large
6'0" to 6'5" (185-95 cm)	30 inches (75 cm)	Extra large
Over 6'5" (195 cm)	33 inches (85 cm)	Extra, extra large

WHAT IS THE BENEFIT?

Life is a balancing act. Our bodies are a complex system of checks and balances. When we get in an off-balance situation, the brain is already sending messages to the neurotransmitters to correct the problem in split-second time. We take this phenomenon for granted. If we play basketball, football, soccer, or tennis or surf, ski, or pursue any other sport that demands us to shift directions at a moment's notice, the body and mind work simultaneously at every moment.

The first day I worked out in the gym with a stability ball, the silent ridicule was deafening. All the credentials in the world couldn't convince the others of the benefits of this simple spherical object. "You'll never catch me on that," or, "That's for girls," were the most popular lines. Or the obvious, "I use that for abs."

So in my infinite wisdom, I got down to the gritty challenge, something everyone understands. Just sitting on the "big ball" drew the attention from most people training in the gym. It made me feel like a circus performer. But it did arouse people's curiosity, and some brave souls took the bait. Suddenly there was silence in the room because everyone knew the extent of what it can do. It all looks easy, and I made it look as though a four-year-old could do it.

As we get older, response times get rusty. The big idea behind the ball is to get your body in an unstable environment. This is where the link between mind and body connect, where small stabilizer muscles tense and release to maintain positioning on the ever-changing curved surface. We never use just one muscle in this routine. We utilize multitudes of them, plus brain power. This gives new meaning to Newton's laws of motion. Whether sitting or lying on the ball, you must be in control. The biggest and best of the muscle groups used are the abdominals and the lower back.

Teaching clients that they have the capacity to do dumbbell presses, ab crunches, leg curls, or squat thrusts on the ball's surface brings a whole new dimension to traditional training. Walking, talking, and chewing gum at the same time isn't so scary anymore! The benefits are endless. Many rehabilitation centers use the ball for several different forms of treatment; professional athletic teams work routines around it training for agility, coordination, and honing the sense of knowing where your body is in space.

Some fitness facilities hold sculpting classes for the young and not-so-young. As ridiculous as a big beach ball looks in a gym, it more than serves its purpose. *Anyone* can use one; some balls can hold up to two thousand pounds. Depending on your height, weight, or skill level, there is a ball for you. They can be used at home or in your office. The cost is low, and with free weights or resistance bands, you've got yourself a great portable gym.

WHEN SHOULD YOU EXPECT TO SEE RESULTS?

You will see results depending on your consistency in as little as four to six weeks. The important thing here is the way you feel. Your posture will improve in a matter of two weeks, and the awareness that you gain in your form and technique will trickle into every aspect of your training routine.

DEFINITIONS AT A GLANCE

Bridge on the Floor. Body positioned on the floor, hips lifted with feet up on the ball.

Bridge on the Ball. Body positioned on the ball, hips lifted with feet on the floor.

Supine. Any exercise set in a position on the ball facing upward.

Prone. Any exercise set in a position on the ball facing downward.

Recline. Sitting in an incline position on the ball, hips lower than the upper body.

Three-position. In Bridge on the Ball, one head plus two shoulders on the ball equals three.

HOW CAN I DO IT RIGHT? THE PROGRAMMING.

Think of standing on the ball as the light at the end of the tunnel. This is possible. Standing is the final frontier. Think of the balance that is required for sitting on the ball first. Multiply that by a hundred. That is how difficult standing on the ball is. In my group classes, I have been able to get people to balance on their hands and knees on top of the ball, and even a few up onto their knees, but standing is the highest level of balance without the application of hand weights, and I have even seen that! Let's get back to warming up.

The Universal Warm-up can be applied to any of the training strategies in this book. Each of the stretches will provide you with enough movement and preparation for strength training at every level, preparation for core training, and flexibility. It applies to any cardiovascular training that you're doing as well. It takes less than ten minutes and will definitely get you going.

UNIVERSAL WARM-UP

WARMING UP. Start your heart by moving for a minimum of five minutes. It doesn't matter if you run in place, jog in place, ride a stationary bike, run up the stairs in your building, or jump rope. Do whatever's available to get your heart and lungs working and joints ready to support you.

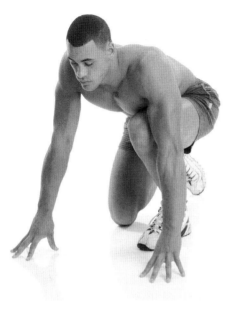

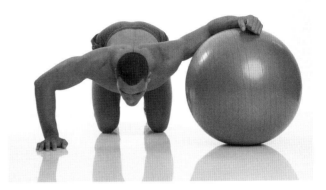

RUNNERS STANCE (HAMSTRING AND LOWER BACK). Imagine you are a sprinter in the Olympics. With your hands touching the floor in front of you, kneel down so one knee touches the floor; the other foot stays directly under your chest. Keeping your torso engaged and your abs firm, lift up through your front leg, raising your hips into the air until you feel the back of your front leg stretch. Hold this position for two seconds and then lower your hips back to the beginning position. Repeat this movement ten times, moving slowly and evenly. Switch to the other leg and repeat.

L-SHAPE CHEST STRETCH (CHEST AND SHOULDER) From the floor, position your body as if you were going to do a modified push-up with your knees on the floor behind you. Using the stability ball as an active way to stretch will help you focus on your shoulders and chest simultaneously. Take the ball under the forearm of one arm, positioning the ball at chest level to your side. Slowly lower your upper body down toward the floor as if you're performing a push-up, feeling the tension in your pectorals and front shoulder muscles. Hold the lower position for two seconds and press yourself back up to the starting position. The ball should stay in place so avoid rolling it from side to side. Repeat the stretch ten times on each arm.

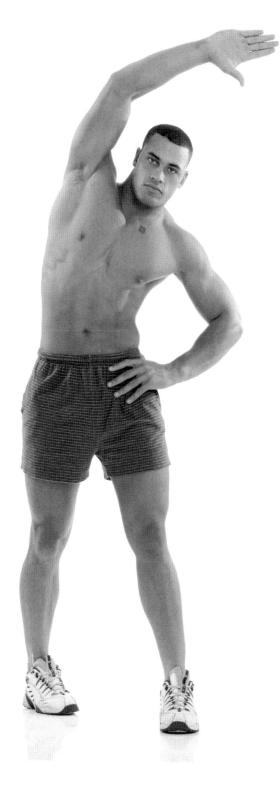

HIP FLEXOR C-CURVE STRETCH (BACK AND FRONT HIP). Standing with your feet a hip's distance apart, shift one leg behind you, keeping the space between your feet the same. Internally rotate your toes so that your heel is pushed to the outside while maintaining heel contact with the floor. Reach into the air with the arm that is on the same side of your body as your back leg, holding the other hand on your waist. Reach up and over to create a C-curve through the middle of you body. You will feel the tension in your obliques and in front of your hips. When lifting your arm up, inhale to assist the expansion of your chest. Reach over ten times, pausing slightly when you reach the C-curve, and then pull your arm back to your side as if you were pulling something with force. Exhale while flexing your lats and biceps as you hit the low end of the contraction. Switch to the other side and repeat.

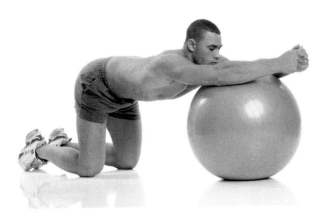

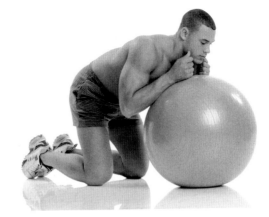

STABILITY BALL
EXERCISES

UPPER BODY

CHEST

LAT PULL ON THE BALL (UNDER ARM, SIDES OF THE BACK AND CORE). From the floor, position your body as if you were going to do a modified push-up with your knees on the floor behind you. The ball is in front of you with both arms resting on it. You should feel your body weight shift forward, rolling the ball forward in order for your abs to engage and your shoulders to stabilize your upper body. You should feel your body weight leaning forward, but not to rest. Pull only your arms back, bending at the elbows in order to engage your back muscles and prep your shoulders. Your arms will stay close to your side, almost touching your body. Inhale as you extend your body over the ball and exhale when you draw your arm in. Repeat ten times, concentrating on the two-second hold at full body extension.

INCLINE AND FLAT CHEST PRESS ON BALL (CHEST AND GLUTES). From a seated position on the ball, walk forward—rolling forward with the ball—holding onto a pair of hand weights. The position of your hips will determine what part of your chest will be the focal point of the exercise. If your hips are parallel to the floor like a tabletop, you are in the flat (bridge) position; your hips being lower than the rest of your body offers you the incline (recline) position. Some people find that the variations provide an option for anyone who experiences lower back pain. The incline version of this illustration will target the upper part of the chest whereas the flat version will target the middle part of your chest. Your upper shoulder area on the ball has to be correct as well. Your shoulder blades should remain pulled together slightly and in contact with the ball for both positions. In the flat position, your head and both shoulders should be resting on the ball. I like to call this the three-point position on the ball. Press both weights

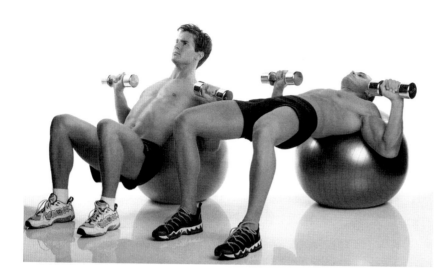

Incline and Flat Chest Press on Ball 2

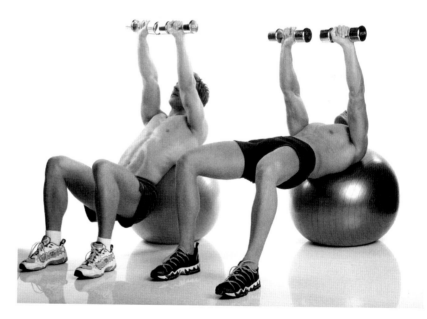

evenly above your chest, bringing your hands together in the top position. With a slow and controlled momentum, lower the weights to chest level in three counts, inhaling as you lower them. Hold for two seconds and exhale as you press back up.

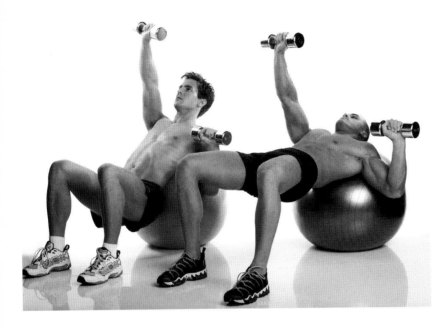

UNILATERAL CHEST PRESS ON BALL (CHEST AND GLUTES). Using the same directions as in the Incline and Flat Chest Press, you will perform a similar exercise with the same setup, but here you will work unilaterally (one arm at a time). The cause and effect will feel very different from the chest press because of the uneven weight that your arms are moving down and up. As you lower each of the hand weights, your torso and the rest of your body has to rethink how to stabilize and not fall off. Breathe in on the lowering of the weight and exhale as you press. Use the same momentum and holds as in the chest press.

FEET ON BALL PUSH-UP (CHEST, SHOULDERS, AND ABS). Standing behind the ball, place your hands on it. Push the ball away from you, rolling your arms onto the ball, then diving out over the ball as you would if you were diving into a lake. Stop when the ball is at your hips and both your feet and hands are touching the floor. From this point, the intensity of the push-up is determined by how far away you position the ball from your center (navel to groin). Walk out lifting one hand at a time, as you did at camp during wheelbarrow races, until you feel you are at a level that suits you. This photo (page 73) illustrates a moderate-to-advanced-level push-up. You can keep the ball under your hips or at midthigh, at knee level, or as shown here, at your ankles. Your hands should be placed at chest level and at about shoulder width. Rotating the position of your hands will affect the chest as well and may be more comfortable depending on your anatomy. Keeping your midsection braced and ready for the exercise, lower your upper body down to about three inches off the floor while breathing in. Hold for a two-second pause and exhale as you press back up. The intensity will also vary depending on the position of your feet. If you bring your body out all the way so that your toes are the only part of your body resting on the ball, to advance the level, allow only your toes to rest. For the most advanced position, take one foot off the ball and hold the extended leg above the ball an inch or so.

HANDS ON BALL PUSH-UP (CHEST AND ABS). Begin with your hands on the ball—positioned with your hands around the edge of the ball, thumbs pointing forward and palms facing in. Your abdominal wall should always be held firm, and your hands should be kept open. As you lower your body, you should inhale as your muscles stretch. The theory behind this type of breathing is that when the space available for the lungs expands, you should fill your lungs with oxygen. As the muscles around your lungs contract, you should expel the air. This makes a lot of sense and offers you a good supply of air as you work. The force of the exhale can also give you a boost to the top when you get tired. Using your chest muscles, press up, extending your arms and lifting your body off the floor. That is one push-up.

Your foot position can also vary depending on how strong you are. If you want to advance the level of the difficulty of the push-up, lift one foot off the floor and support the middle section of your body between your hands and your feet. Your buttocks should also be positioned slightly higher than they would be if you were lying on the floor. This simple direction will also keep you aware of your abdominal position.

Your head should extend naturally off your shoulders, and your eyes should be fixed on the floor beneath you. This will help you to focus and stay in the exercise.

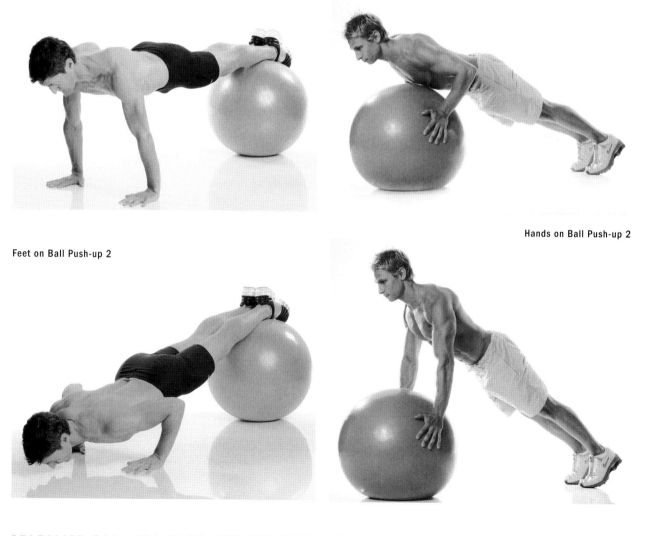

Feet on Ball Push-up 1

Hands on Ball Push-up 1

Feet on Ball Push-up 2

Hands on Ball Push-up 2

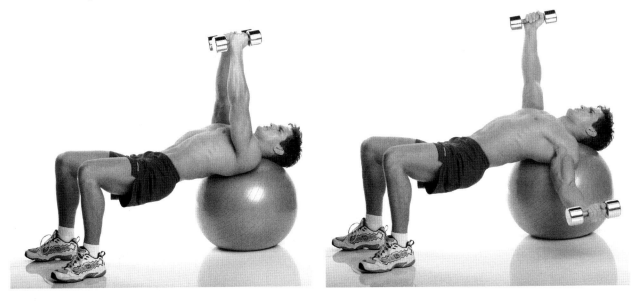

UNILATERAL BALL FLYE (CHEST AND GLUTES) Sit down on the ball and rest your hand weights on your knees until you are ready to begin. Walk forward—rolling forward with the ball—holding onto a pair of hand weights with caution, resting the weights until you are flat and in the bridge position. Bring one dumbbell in by bending your arm at the elbow and holding the weight at your chest and then the other weight to your chest as well. Extend both arms up, lifting the dumbbells over your chest and keeping your elbows bent. With your palms facing each other, you are ready to begin the ball flyes.

Imagine your arms are wrapped around a barrel, creating a rounded position with the weight above. As you lower each dumbbell down toward the floor by slowly opening each arm out to the side independently of the other, feel the pulling of your chest muscles on the outer side of the chest, where your shoulders and chest interconnect. This is the all-important stretch you need to feel in order to challenge the muscle to get stronger. When the weight is lower than your body, stop and press the weight back up to the starting position. Your torso and the rest of your body have to renegotiate your balance and figure out how to stabilize so you don't fall off. Concentrate on feeling the inside part of your chest as you raise and lower the weight against gravity. By doing so, you are always present in the exercise, and the performance gets a better reaction from the muscles.

BALL PULL OVER (LATS, OBLIQUES, AND GLUTES) The setup is safer than just getting on the ball and picking up a set of weights. Try to establish good habits. Sit down on the ball and rest your hand weights on your knees until you are ready to begin. Walk forward—rolling forward with the ball—holding onto a pair of hand weights with caution, resting the weights until you are flat and in the bridge position. Bring each weight into the air above your chest with your palms facing forward. Keeping your buttocks muscles engaged and the weight of your body supported from your abs, lower your arms back toward the floor slowly as you inhale. It is important not to arch your back up into the air. Hold your body position as rigidly as you can.

Ball Preacher Curl 1

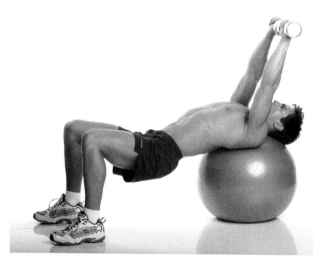

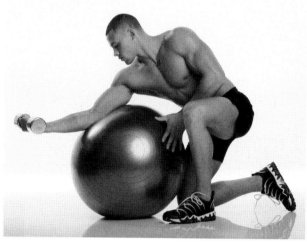

Ball Pull Over 2

Ball Preacher Curl 2

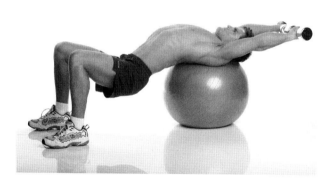

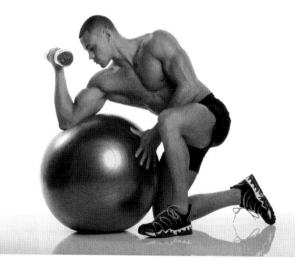

ARMS

To begin the Pull Over, pull your abs in by emphasizing the drawing of your ribs toward your pelvis. This pull will automatically fire up the muscles leading to your arms, helping your arms pull back into their starting position. As you pull, you should exhale. All of these support moves are what will make a difference when you train on a traditional weight bench.

BALL PREACHER CURL (BICEPS). Kneel down on the floor with the ball in front of you. Bring one leg to the side of the ball and position the other leg behind you touching the ball. Bring your upper body forward by bending at the waist. Put one hand down, grab a dumbbell off the floor, and rest your free hand on the back of the ball. With the arm that is holding the

Seated Ball Biceps Curl 1

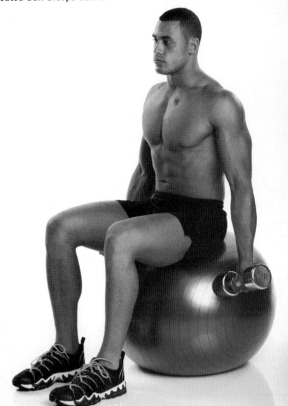

weight, stabilize your elbow against the top of ball on the same side of the body as your knee. Don't let it move or slide around; keep it resting on the ball at all times during this exercise. Bend your elbow and bring the weight up to your shoulders, and squeeze your biceps tight. Hold for a second, and then lower the weight back down slowly. After a few reps, you will feel how difficult this isolated curl really is. Repeat until you reach your set and then move to the other arm.

SEATED BALL BICEPS CURL (BICEPS). This classic exercise concentrates on the front of the arms. Sit with your feet apart, about shoulder width, stabilizing through your legs and torso. Remember that your feet position will regulate the intensity level as well as the weight choice for all the exercises. Hold a dumbbell in each hand with your palms facing forward. Try to contain the movement of your body as you lift and lower the dumbbells from their start and finish positions. Bending both arms at the same time until your hands face the front of your shoulders, bring the weight up to shoulder level. Add a short pause at the top of the contraction, then lower the weight back down slowly to hip level and repeat. You can also alternate each arm (as with the unilateral presses described in the chest and shoulder exercises) until you have completed a full set of single repetitions for each arm.

Seated Ball Biceps Curl 2

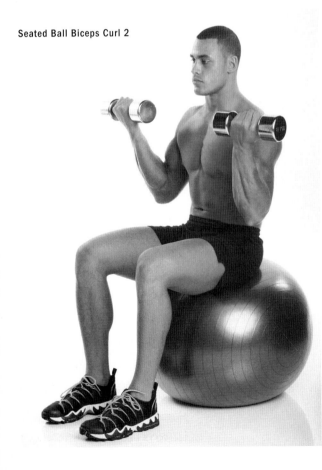

ON THE BALL TRICEPS EXTENSIONS "SKULL CRUSHERS" (TRICEPS). This exercise requires astute awareness of your body position and spine support. Choose a low weight that will allow you to learn the best technique to best isolate the back of your arm. Once you grasp the importance of form, you can move on to greater gains.

Position your weight on the ball. Walk forward—rolling forward with the ball—holding onto your hand

On the Ball Triceps Extensions 1

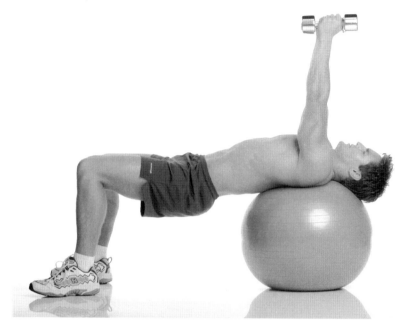

On the Ball Triceps Extensions 2

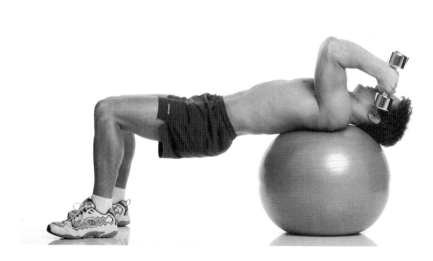

firm midsection, and stay parallel to the floor in your bridge position. Anchor your shoulders as you lift and lower the weights, holding onto the three-point position against the ball. It could be dangerous to throw your body into the momentum. If you are using your body this way, consider lowering the weight of your dumbbells.

BALL DIPS (TRICEPS). I still consider the triceps to be the sexiest muscles of the body. It seems as though they do more than their share of work; and when you need to work these muscles, you need to work them hard. An ideal way to give your triceps the challenge and overload they need to become impressive is by using your own body as the weight they need to fatigue. This is one of those exercises that requires you to be fearless and step out of your comfort zone. You have to fight falling off the ball at the same time you are trying to do the exercise. Exercises that require you to support your own body weight are perfect for travel, and this is one of them.

Sit on the ball with your hands resting at your sides. Put your hands beside your hips and place them palm down on the ball. Your fingers should be positioned forward, to stabilize your hands from slipping. If

weights until you are in the three-point bridge position. Bring your arms up one at a time into the air and establish your set position. Allow your arms to drift back slightly to engage the back of both arms and feel your triceps activate. Lower the hand weights in the

same three-countdown, two-second hold and then press the weights up by extending your arms fully, carrying the weight above you until you feel your arms flex completely. Hold on for a moment and then slowly release down to the start position and repeat. Maintain a

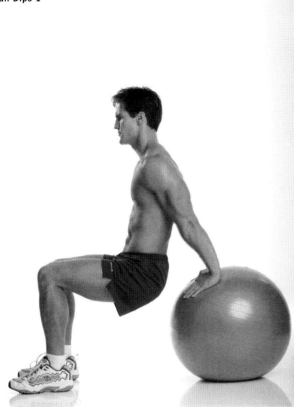

you need to change the position to suit your wrist stabilizers, go ahead and find your position. Lift your body weight off the ball with your arms and shoulder strength and contract your abs for a secure position. It is important for you to keep your shoulders down and away from your ears. Shift your weight forward away from the hips and away from the ball about two inches or so. No more than that. You do not want this to go to your shoulders. With your feet flat on the floor in front of you, slowly bend your elbows, lowering your erect torso down toward the floor. You should resemble an elevator cab moving up and down a shaft rather than an escalator that moves diagonally. Isolate your triceps while maintaining your arm position directly behind you, not flared out to the side.

Focus your eyes in front of you as you press up through the back of the arms and as you reach the top. Hold your shoulders down away from your ears at all times. Repeat your set number of reps and continue.

SHOULDERS

BALL SEATED FORWARD SHOULDER RAISE (ANTERIOR DELTS). This exercise targets the anterior (front) shoulder. As with the overhead press, body position and foot placement are key elements for best results and execution. Hold your abs firm and feel the support for the spine, especially the lower part. Foot position is up to you—remember that the closer your feet are, the more difficult the exercise becomes. Feet can rest on the floor either separated about shoulder width or closer together. Knees should always stay at a 90-degree bend, so that your feet are positioned directly beneath your knees.

Focus directly ahead of you at a spot on the wall and inhale. Holding the dumbbells, keep your thumbs

Ball Dips 2

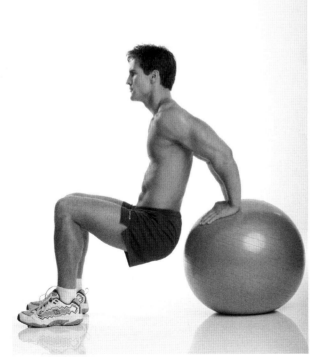

Ball Seated Forward Shoulder Raise

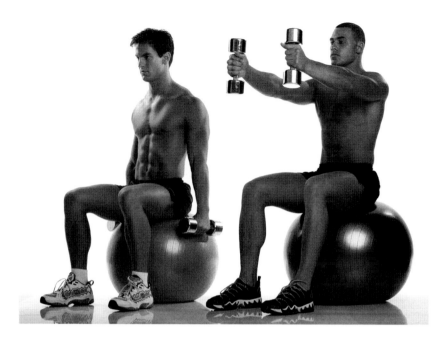

Ball Seated Lateral Raise

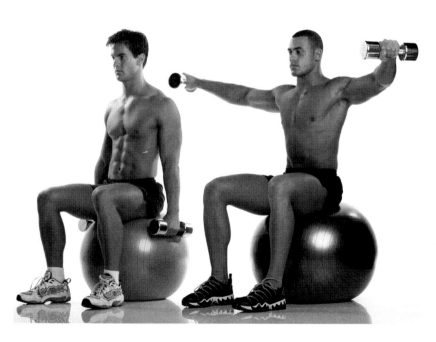

and then switch to the other side. Try not to race. Give the process time and concentrate on executing it perfectly every time.

In a duo raise, you lift both dumbbells at the same time. Vary the same exercise by performing the front raise one arm at a time as we did with some of the chest exercises. Pay attention to the way the dumbbells move through space, and make sure you have control over them and that they're not leading you.

Internally and externally rotating your shoulders can offer variety as well. Internally rotated means that your thumbs are pointing in. One negative to internal rotation is its overuse. Internally rotated exercises are performed routinely, and the movement is repeated in daily tasks. By externally rotating your shoulders (thumbs position forward) with the dumbbells, you have opened the shoulders and relieved pinning of the front shoulders, which is common. If you are just beginning a weight-training program, any of the exercises targeting the front shoulders are fine, and you should continue with the appropriate weight and sets.

pointing forward and arms resting at your sides. Exhale as you lift each dumbbell forward. Lift each hand, carrying the weight to about shoulder level directly in front of you, no higher. You are working against gravity, so don't expect this to be easy. Lower the weight slowly

BALL SEATED LATERAL RAISE (MEDIAL DELTS). The lateral raise will broaden your shoulders and give you that swimmer's build that

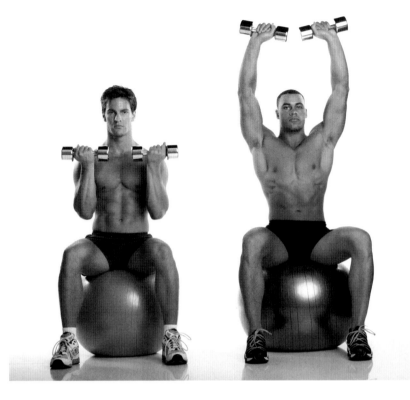

so many men want. The *medial deltoid,* or cap of the shoulder, may require you to use lighter weights than you might be using for the other exercises. This doesn't mean that you should reduce the weights so much that you can't feel anything or lift such a heavy load that your technique suffers. Monitor yourself and make an effort to promote strength behind the form.

Keep the weights at or just below the shoulders. Sit with your feet apart, and your midsection braced. Your chest should stay lifted and your arms extended, with a slight bend at the elbow. Holding onto your dumbbells with your palms facing in toward your body,

pointing your thumbs in front of you, focus straight ahead and begin by lifting the weights outward with a slow and controlled lift. Lift the weights to about shoulder height and then stop and hold for a moment while your arms are parallel to the floor. Using the exhale to assist the lift will help ensure that you aren't throwing your body weight into the exercise. Lower the weights slowly and feel the outside of your shoulders as you ease it down. You can also rotate your thumbs upward to externally rotate the shoulders as a variation. Repeat the lateral raise for as many repetitions as desired for the set and then rest.

BALL SEATED OVERHEAD SHOULDER PRESS. This exercise will concentrate on the front, sides, and back of your shoulders simultaneously. This particular exercise is wonderful because it takes care of three muscles at once. Individual hand weights require you to think about where the weights are in space. It determines independent motion as a technical skill and promotes natural rotation of the shoulder at the same time.

Support the weights at shoulder height with arms gripped at shoulder width. Your hands should be turned in to face your shoulders. Your feet should stabilize on the floor in front of you in a position

Ball Hyperextension 1

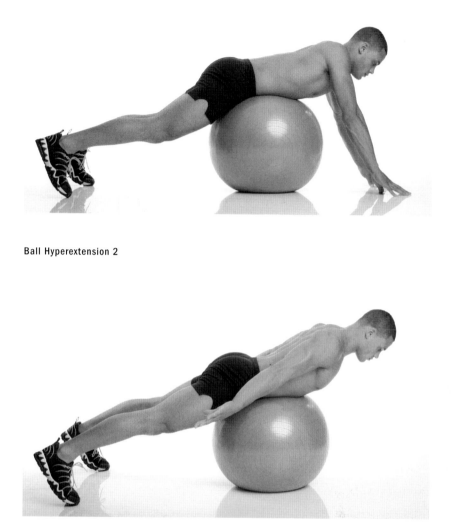

Ball Hyperextension 2

that suits your level of balance. Keep your gut tight and avoid arching your back when you have the weights above your head (or at any other time, for that matter). Maintain a neutral grip of your hands, meaning hands over wrists, wrists over elbows, to prevent stress on the wrists and ensure better form.

Press the weights up into the air, exhaling as you do, with a smooth and deliberate contraction.

The rotation takes place in the action of the press up, not at the top of the contraction. As your hands reach the midpoint of pressing into the air, turn them to face front. Avoid pushing the weights forward and then up; the stress of that action could be dangerous. Hold the weights above your head for a short stop and then lower the weights downward slowly, again with a deliberate, controlled motion. Repeat

the set number of reps and the number of sets.

BALL HYPEREXTENSIONS. Begin in a prone position on the ball with your hands and feet evenly placed on either side of it. Hips and stomach are on the ball, balls of the feet are on the floor, keeping your head extended from your shoulders in one line with your spine. Begin by pulling the navel toward the spine

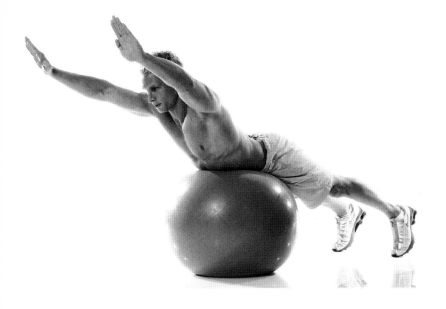

to engage your abdominals. This is very similar to a traditional push-up position, but in this exercise you have a ball under your hips to support your body weight. Gently squeeze the glutes and the hamstrings, keeping your eyes focused on the floor. Inhale and slowly extend your back, lifting your upper body away from the ball from the chest. Your arm movements will rotate back, similar to a swim stroke. I always tell my clients to imagine paddling a surfboard or swimming the breast stroke. The move should have the same feel to it—controlled. As you sweep the arms back, feel the retraction of your shoulder blades, which should now be active, and hold your position steady. Do not hyperextend your spine. Also, try not to shift your gaze to the ceiling to avoid flexing your neck. Hold the upper position for two seconds. Exhale slowly as you return to your starting position. Repeat ten to twelve times for a complete set. If your feet slip, place the soles of your feet against the wall.

UPPER BODY HYPEREXTENSIONS

Similar to the ball hyperextensions, this exercise requires you to trust your balance enough to lift both arms as in the illustration. Assume a prone body position on the ball with your hands and feet evenly placed on either side of it. Roll back slightly to give your lower body some leverage, just enough to feel as though you can lift your hands off the floor. Keep your eyes focused on the floor until you start to lift off the ball. Start lifting with your arms extended, making this action the initial part of the contraction. Inhale as you lift your upper body with control. Your shoulders will be less likely to retract, but they should feel as if they are pressing or sliding down toward your lower back and glutes. In fact, the upper buttocks area should feel the stabilizing effect of this exercise more than anywhere else. Repeat ten to twelve reps per set.

LOWER BODY

LEGS

BALL WALL SQUAT (QUADS AND GLUTES) This exercise can be performed with either your body

Ball Wall Squat 1

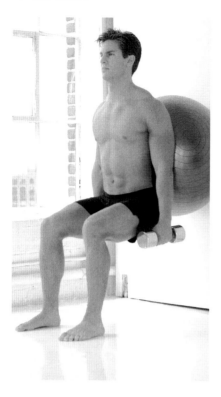

Ball Wall Squat 2

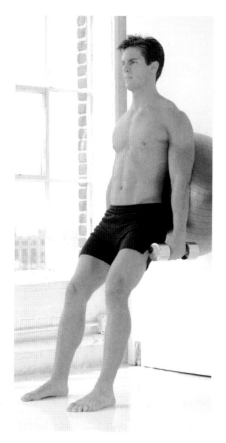

weight only or with a set of dumbbells. If using weights to add intensity, choose weights for your level and remember that this is a large muscle group that might require heavier weights in order to overload. This exercise will utilize all the muscles of the lower body collectively, the quadriceps, hamstrings, and glutes (butt), which are three separate muscles—gluteus maximus, gluteus minimus, and gluteus medius—as well as all muscles in the torso. Your lower back and abdominal region (core) must participate in order to support the exercise. This exercise requires focus, balance, and serious attention to technique in order to be be effective.

If you are using dumbbells, hold the weights in both hands next to your hips, directly below your shoulders with your arms relaxed. If you are not using weights, keep your hands at your sides.

Position your feet hip distance apart with your toes turned out just slightly. Keep your chest lifted in a natural postural position with your eyes looking directly in front of you and your chin pulled in slightly. As you sit down, roll the ball downward against the wall while lowering your body weight. The weight of your body and the weights you are carrying should be

felt in your legs and buttocks. You want to come down slowly, imagining that there is a chair underneath for you to sit on. Stop when your knees reach a 90-degree angle. Inhale as you bring the weights down, and work with slow, controlled momentum. Lower the dumbbells as if you are putting them on the floor, maintaining your perfect posture. When you lower the weights, the tendency is to bend forward. This tip should remind you to sit back and keep your chest lifted. Exhale as you press upward to the starting position and feel the heels of your feet pushing the load through your legs. Stay off the balls of the feet to take stress off your knees. If you feel pressure in the knees, lighten the weights or remove them completely. Practice by sitting down in a hardwood chair and standing up again repeatedly until you understand the range of motion and the muscles used in the exercise. Just touch your buttocks down on the chair lightly and then stand up again. Keep repeating until you get it right, then you will be ready to squat using the ball and weights.

FLOOR BRIDGE (HAMSTRINGS, GLUTES, AND ABS). Starting on the floor may mislead you into thinking that this is an easy exer-

Floor Bridge

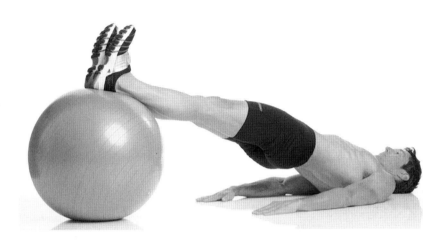

Floor Bridge Hip Rotations

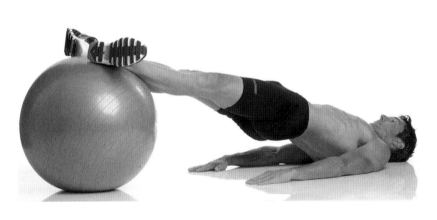

cise. Think again. Lie down on the floor with your feet resting on top of the ball at around the heel and lowest half of your calves. Try positioning your feet about two inches away from each other to give you additional balance. This position is named the Floor Bridge and will be used for several exercises throughout this book.

Focus your eyes above you as you inhale. Exhale as you lift your body off the floor from the hips, using your glutes to lift. The exhalation will pull your abdominals in against your spine in order to support your back. When you reach the point where your body resembles a plank, stop and hold. You should maintain a comfortable shoulder position so you don't stress the back of your neck. Lower yourself back to the floor with a slow and controlled momentum, resting slightly at floor level. Repeat until you finish the required number of reps. If you want to intensify further, after you have perfected your technique, try extending both arms into the air above your chest toward the ceiling. This will force maximum effort of your entire lower body and challenge your balance skill.

FLOOR BRIDGE HIP ROTATIONS (HAMSTRINGS, GLUTES, INNER AND OUTER THIGHS). Lie down on the floor with your feet resting on top of the ball at around your heels and lowest half of your calves. The exercise is very similar to the Floor Bridge, with an added component. Lift the lower body into the air by contracting the glutes and the abs to get you into the supine plank position. When you reach the desired height, when you feel as though your buttocks are engaged and you are fully extended, hold and rotate your toes outward to the side. Hold that rotation for a second while you squeeze your buttocks together and then rotate your toes back to the upright position. When you finish the single rotation, relax slowly back down to the floor and repeat.

Single Leg Floor Bridge

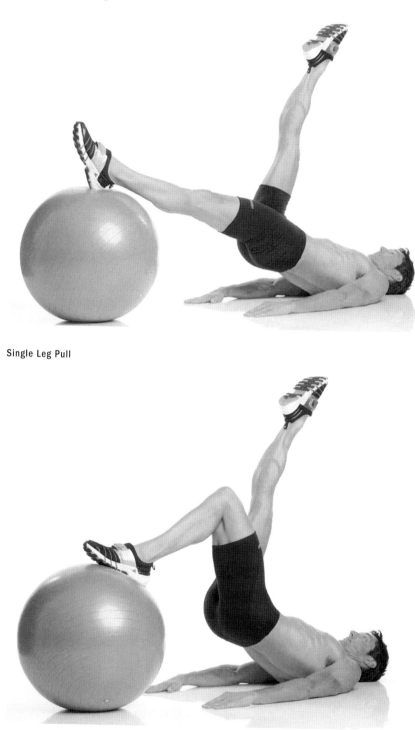

Single Leg Pull

from the hips, using your glutes to raise yourself off the floor. The exhalation will pull your abdominals in against your spine in order to support your back. When you reach the point where your body resembles a plank, stop and hold. You should maintain a comfortable shoulder position so you don't stress the back of your neck.

The challenge here is to lift one fully extended leg off the ball. Lift the leg with a controlled motion and be sure not to rush into the position as you will lose your balance. You want to extend the leg by pulling your thigh and the abdominal muscles in toward the spine. Point your toe to ensure full extension of your leg. Slowly bring the extended leg back down to the ball and relax your entire body to the floor for relief. Repeat on the other side, alternating each leg.

SINGLE LEG PULL. Lie down on the floor with your feet resting on top of the ball at around the heels and lowest half of your calves. Focus your eyes above you as you inhale. Exhale and lift up into the supine bridge position with your body maintaining a neutral position, both heels on the ball and shoulders on the floor. Your arms should be kept to the sides for sup-

SINGLE LEG FLOOR BRIDGE (HAMSTRINGS, GLUTES, AND ABS). Lie down on the floor with your feet resting on top of the ball at around the heels and lowest half of your calves. Focus your eyes above you as you inhale. Exhale as you lift your body off the floor

port. Lift one fully extended leg off the ball into the Single Leg Floor Bridge position. Keep your remaining leg on the exercise ball and pull your heel toward your hips, rolling the ball along the floor while keeping the suspended leg rigid. Try to keep your hips as neutral as possible, allowing most of the movement to come from your bent leg. Repeat with the other leg.

Ball Crunch 1

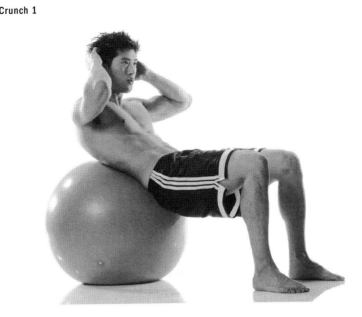

CORE ONLY

Ball Crunch 2

BALL CRUNCH This is the most common exercise that you see people perform on the stability ball. An exerciser can create a greater range of motion than is possible on a flat surface, which forces your abdominal area to stretch farther than it normally does. Start by sitting on the ball with a comfortable foot stance. Keeping your hands on the ball beside your hips, walk out to your recline position, keeping your hips slightly lower than your upper body. The ball should be resting at midback with your lower back touching the ball at the top of your buttocks. With your hands held behind your head—separated, not laced together—lift your upper body away from the ball with an even exhalation. Try tilting your

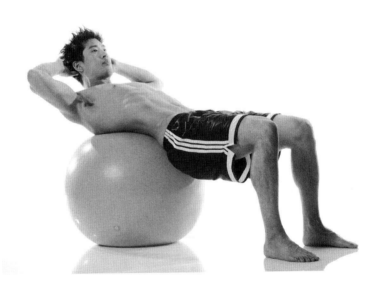

chin down just slightly without cocking your head back and forth as you lift up off the ball. The abdominal muscles will roll your spine off the ball, and the beginning of that rolling effort should come from your head and travel down toward your pelvis.

BALL ROMAN TWIST. Start by sitting on the ball with a comfortable foot stance. Keeping your hands on the ball beside your hips, walk out to your recline position keeping your hips slightly lower than your upper body. The ball should be resting at midback with your lower

Ball Roman Twist 1

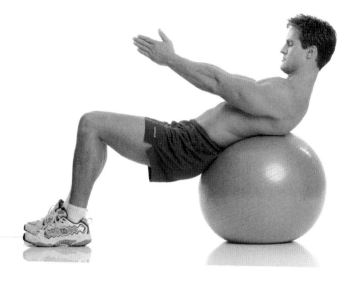

Ball Roman Twist 2

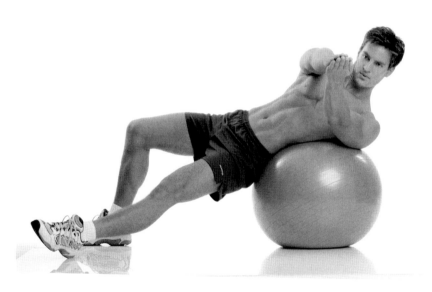

back touching the ball at the top of your buttocks. Tilt your butt slightly to engage the glutes and pull your navel in. Instead of holding your hands behind your head, bring them together as if you were going to dive into a pool, pointing toward the top corner of the room. With your upper body already supported in a semicrunch contraction, rotate your upper and lower body to one side. As you roll to that side, you have to extend your leg on the same side completely in order not to fall. You should rotate in a slow and controlled manner, keeping your eyes focused on your hands. You will have to put on the brakes when you finally reach the side and stop completely. Then lift your hands back to the starting position and over to the other side without stopping midway. Make sure you put on your brakes to stop the rotation. This exercise may not feel like a traditional ab exercise, but the benefits are huge.

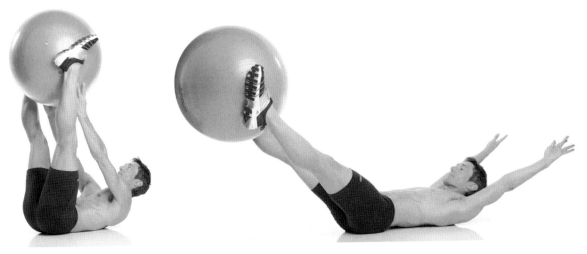

Ball Switch 2

Ball Switch 3

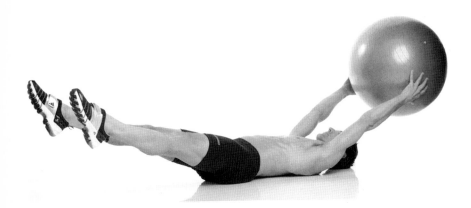

BALL SWITCH (UPPER TO LOWER). This exercise is highly advanced. Practice it without the ball first, and as you become stronger and more precise, add the ball. Follow the description, just leave the ball to the side at least the first few times you do it. Start by lifting your feet into the air with your legs fully extended and raise your arms up to touch your feet while your shoulders lift off the floor to help you reach your goal. With a slow and controlled movement, let your arms and legs slowly lower toward to the floor, extending your body completely. Stop when your legs are about four or five inches from the floor. You will feel a tremendous effect here in the middle of your body. From that fully extended supine position on the floor, tighten your torso, and lift both your legs and arms at the same time to meet at the top. Repeat.

Using the ball adds a heightened intensity to an already difficult exercise. Hold the ball between your hands as you extend on the

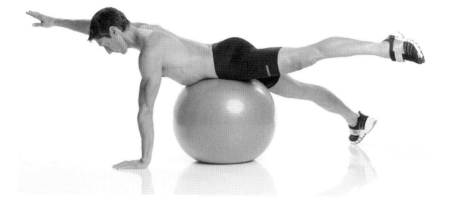

floor. Lifting both your legs and arms along with the ball, meet in the middle and exchange the ball so that it is held between your feet. You will hold the ball isometrically between your feet just as you did with your hands as you lower the ball toward the floor with your legs. Stop before the ball touches the floor and begin the cycle again. You will need the power of breath here to ensure that you are holding with the center of your body and not antagonizing your lower back. If at any time this exercise feels too extreme, put the ball down and stop.

SWIMMER. Begin in a prone position on the ball with your hands and feet evenly placed on either side of the ball. Hips and stomach are on the ball, balls of your feet are on the floor, keeping your head extended from your shoulders in one line with your spine. Begin by pulling your navel toward your spine to engage the abdominals. This is very similar to a traditional push-up position, but here you have a ball under your hips to support your body weight. Gently squeeze your glutes and hamstrings, keeping your eyes directed to the floor. Independently lift your arms and legs to perform this exercise. You have done this on the floor before. Understand that as you exert your body, your brain must make an effort also. With your midsection braced lift your right hand as if you were raising it to ask a question. At the same time elevate your left leg off the floor using your butt muscles. You want to feel the contraction diagonally across the middle of your back using your shoulders, middle back, and upper buttocks. Slowly release back to the original position and switch to the opposite hand and foot. Make sure you have a wider than shoulder-width hand position on the floor to give you better leverage.

LOWER BODY HYPERS. Starting on the ball in the prone position, with the ball under your sternum, bend your elbows enough to get your upper body positioned slightly lower than the top of the ball. Your hands will have to separate slightly wider than shoulder width and it may help to turn your fingers in slightly for balance. Your toes should be resting on the floor at this point. Tighen your butt muscles together and feel your legs lift into the air. Keeping your legs ex-

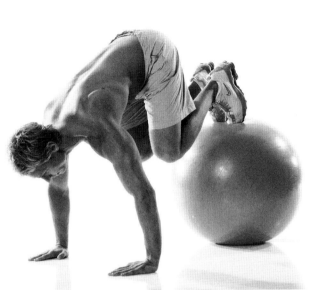

Ball Pike

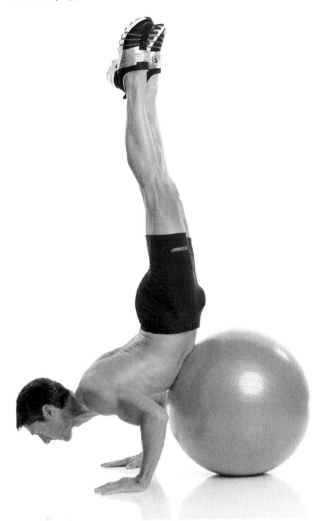

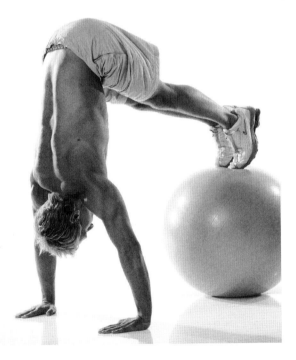

tended, exhale as you lift both legs up as high as you feel comfortable. This may be an inch off the floor, even with the floor, or slightly higher. Work within your own fitness level. The photograph illustrates an advanced level for this exercise, which is can also be considered a shoulder stand. Reach full extension, hold for two seconds, and lower back down slowly. As with many of the exercises in this book, the interest in containing the movement is vital and loaded with benefits. Repeat this exercise ten to twelve reps per set.

BALL TUCK. Think of tucking your knees into your chest. Starting in the push-up position, place your feet and shins on the ball and your palms on the floor, hands aligned under your shoulders. Remember that the placement of the ball is important for intensity levels. If the ball were resting at thigh level, this exercise would feel easier and there would be less stress put on your hands, wrists, and shoulders. Start the Ball Tuck by bending your legs, pulling the ball toward your upper body, keeping the focus on tucking your abs in as you curl inward. Exhale as you pull in toward your upper body and control where the ball is rolling. Roll in until you are on your toes, or until you feel you cannot go any farther. The balance between your upper body and your lower body will be challenged. Your abs will not only support the pull but will support the push-up position when you extend. Inhale as you roll back into the starting position. Continue bending your knees until your thighs are close to your chest and your coccyx is pointing toward the ceiling. Release and repeat.

BALL PIKE. Starting on the ball in the push-up position, place your feet and shins on the ball and your palms on the floor, hands aligned under your shoulders. The difference between the tuck and the pike is the level of intensity and how many muscles are used. Perfect the tuck before attempting the pike. That said, the only way to do the pike is to change your footing and start at toe level. Start with the top part of both feet (where the laces of your shoes are) on the ball. In the push-up position, breathe in and prepare for the lift. As you exhale, lift your coccyx or the end of your spine upward into the air. As you lift, the ball will roll toward your hands. Stop when you are at a 90-degree angle. You should not exceed the 90 degrees as you will roll over yourself. Stop when your torso is vertical and your eyes directly facing the ball. Hold for two seconds and roll the ball with your feet back to the push-up position.

Hamstring Stretch

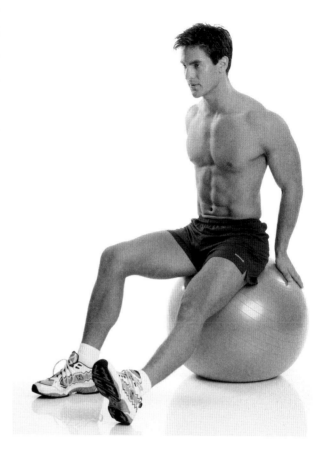

STRETCHES

HAMSTRING STRETCH. Sit with good posture on the ball. Rolling forward slightly, extend your right leg in front of you, with your shoe heels on the floor, toes flexed up and pulled back toward your upper body. To intensify this stretch, start by placing your hands behind you with your fingers turned to the back of the room. Roll the ball slightly until you feel the ball tilt your pelvis enough to enhance the stretch. Now bend from the waist, bringing the chest down closer toward your legs. Maintain the extension of your head off your shoulders to prevent a jutting of your chin. This only stresses the neck and upper shoulders, preventing you from getting the benefit of the stretch. Try to re-

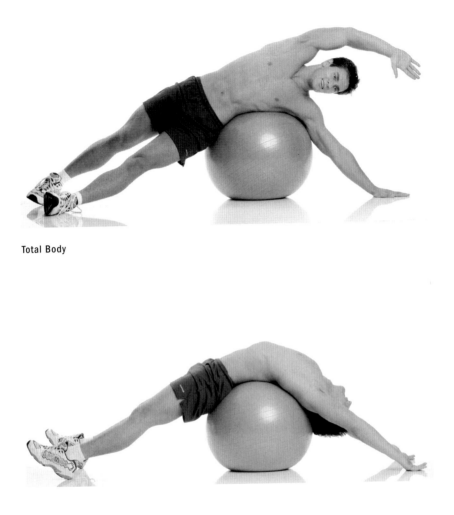

Total Body

lax your face with each stretch. Release by sitting back on top of the ball and repeat on the other side.

SIDE STRETCH. Starting from a seated position, roll forward first into the supine position on the ball. Roll over and lie on your right side, resting on the ball with your right hip, ribcage, and armpit on the ball. With both legs extended, position your right foot on the floor (outside of the foot against the floor) in front of your left foot (inside of the foot against the floor) for balance. For more stability, touch your right hand to the floor. Extend your left arm overhead and relax. Hold for about ten seconds (or more if you wish) and repeat on the left side.

TOTAL BODY. Start from a supine position on the ball, with the ball placed on the center of your back. Stabilize both of your feet to keep them securely on the floor in front of you. Leading with your arms, power up from the heels of your feet in a slow, controlled fashion, allowing the ball to roll along your spine. This one move should feel really good. Finish the movement when the body is fully extended over the ball. The Total Body is really a supported back bend. If you feel uncomfortable with your head down, don't go so far. If there is any discomfort in the lower back area, roll forward and out of the stretch. Return to the start position in a slow, controlled fashion. You might feel a bit light-headed when you come out of the stretch; this is normal.

ADDITIONAL EXERCISES FOR THE LOWER BODY (WITHOUT THE BALL)

These exercises are being described rather than photographed for a few reasons. First, these three exercises have been seen in every magazine known to man and woman. They are classic exercises and you have probably performed them at one time or another, and finally, they offer an aerobic component that some of the other exercises for the lower body do not. Namely, because you are moving through space, using the entire lower and midsection of the body, your heart has to work harder, pushing your heart rate back into a moderate training mode. I wanted to insert these exercises as options for you to use. Consider using one or all three as part of a warm-up or perform a set of one exercise between sets of strength exercises. Anyway you choose will be a benefit to your routine and boost your training to the next level.

WALKING LUNGE. A personal favorite. Standing tall with your hands at your side, take a giant step forward with what we will call the lead foot, keeping the front knee positioned above the front foot and the back knee bent (much like the warrior yoga pose on page 106). Instead of pushing yourself back to the starting position, continue your forward movement and bring the back foot in to meet the lead foot. You will feel the weight in your front leg as you take these giant steps one after the other, alternating the lead foot with each step. If you have enough space, try to do eight steps down a hallway or try four and then turn around and

do four more. In all, try to do at least sixteen Walking Lunges per set.

LATERAL LUNGE. This lunge will definitely affect your buttocks and inner thighs. From a standing position, take a giant step out to the side, much like the previous exercise described above. You are traveling sideways, so take notice of how your feet are positioned. They should both be pointed directly in front of you. The side-stepping foot will want to angle outward, but try to keep it pointed forward. The step should be wider than your shoulders, and even wider to maximize the exercise. Your upper body needs to stay as upright as possible, avoiding bending too much at the waist. Keeping the braced feeling around your waist will remind you to support the abs, thus supporting the exercise itself. Bend the knee of the leg you stepped out with to a 90-degree angle and push back into your standing position. Repeat twelve times per leg. Intensify the Lateral Lunge by adding hand weights in each hand.

STEP-UPS. You will need a platform or a chair that measures at least six inches to sixteen inches as a prop. Stand about four inches away from the prop with your hands at your side. Lift one foot onto the prop and place it on the prop with the entire sole of the shoe, heel to toe. Climb up to the top of the prop using the buttocks and the leg muscles to carry you up. Maintain a braced midsection to support your spine and keep your eyes looking forward. Climb down using the same foot you started with and lower yourself down back down to the floor. Move with slow and intentional movements and remember not to bounce. Perform fifteen Step-ups for each leg. Intensify the Step-up by adding hand weights.

The Push-up

The Push Away

The Pull Down

The Pull Toward

The Full Extension

THE FAST AND THE FURIOUS

I know that many of you reading this book want the fastest gains possible. Going through each routine in this book once will not give you the body that you want. In the end, it will take time and commitment. It won't happen overnight. Here's why. There are certain muscles that respond faster to weight training than others; some seemingly shape up after one round of the machine circuit. If you want quick, visible proof of your workout, know which body parts to focus on first.

Muscles are classified as "fast twitch" or "slow twitch." Slow-twitch muscles are found in large or stabilizing muscle groups such as the abdomen or back. These muscle fibers can typically contract for long periods of time and are difficult to fatigue, which makes them slow to get defined by exercise.

Fatigue is a signal of overload that stimulates your muscles to adapt by getting stronger. When a muscle fatigues, the central nervous system initiates mechanisms to increase fiber recruitment within the muscle and eventually causes the muscle to hypertrophy (that is, get bigger) to produce more force. This neuromuscular adaptation takes place very rapidly and is why the first few weeks of strength training often yields large increases in strength without any noticeable change in size.

Your stomach muscles, for instance, are slow twitch and basically contract all day long to stabilize the body. Essentially, they have been working out for sixteen-plus hours a day since you were able to sit up by yourself and are therefore in good shape. The downside is that they are difficult to overload during training; *hypertrophy* (the visible gain of muscle definition) comes slowly. Typically, it takes two to three months of regular sit-ups to see any visible change in stomach muscle definition.

The back, on the other hand, has a greater variation of fiber type. The upper back and shoulders respond faster to regular weight training than the stabilizing muscles of the lower back. After four to six weeks of targeted exercises, like military presses, side dumbbell raises, seated rows, and even lat pull downs, you will start to see enhanced muscle tone in your shoulder area. As for the gluteus maximus, which is roughly equally composed of slow- and fast-twitch fibers, results come quickly because you can use larger weights to overload these muscles faster.

Fast-twitch muscles, found in the arms and legs, contract quickly and usually respond better to strength training than slow-twitch fiber muscles because they're easier to overload and fatigue. They will also experience greater increases in size.

Of course, just one session in the weight room won't do the trick. If you've seen bodybuilders doing biceps curls before a competition, they're not trying to get a quick fix of muscle definition. Instead, they're increasing blood flow to the muscles that will definitely cause their arms to look temporarily bigger. Expect substantive results to take at least a few weeks. The difference between how slow-twitch and fast-twitch muscle react explains why it is so difficult to get perfectly cut abs and relatively easy to develop bulging biceps and calves.

THE MEDICINE BALL

WHAT ARE THEY?

If the last time you picked up a medicine ball was in your high school gym class, it's time to take another look at this training tool. Medicine balls today are a departure from the worn leather balls of the past. They're high-tech, colorful, and made with an easy-to-grip rubberized surface.

Modern balls are eons ahead of the old-fashioned leather ones. But do medicine balls measure up to traditional weight machines and dumbbells? Absolutely. With balls ranging from one to fifty pounds, you can work just as hard. In fact, Roland Strong points out that the medicine ball surpasses many other forms of resistance equipment. Medicine balls fill a void that traditional weights can't because they allow you to successfully train using dynamic *and* random movements. That's because today's medicine balls also bounce.

There's no end to the benefits of medicine-ball training. You can use them for developing all major muscles groups in various environments.

HOW DO YOU CHOOSE THE RIGHT ONE?

Medicine balls come in a variety of weights ranging from one to fifty pounds. There are heavier medicine balls out there, but for most purposes I would recommend a ball between three and twelve pounds. They also come in a variety of surfaces from the classic leather style of the old gym days, to the more modern versions that have a rubber coating and bounce. Try a few at the sporting goods store and see which feels best for you.

WHAT IS THE BENEFIT?

1. IMPROVES SPORTS PERFORMANCE. Training with a medicine ball simulates real sports situations and improves hand-eye coordination because you can throw, catch, and bounce it. Tossing or moving with the ball also develops power for sport-specific actions like golf swings, tennis serves, and swimming strokes. And medicine balls are well-suited for *plyometric exercises*—jumping or explosive movements—because they're safer than traditional dumbbells.

2. CHALLENGES YOUR CORE. Tossing and catching a medicine ball improves core strength and stabilization, which decreases the risk of injury and enhances performance. Training with the ball also facilitates functional movement, especially in the torso, so everyday activities are easier and safer. For instance, doing spinal rotations with the ball mimics lifting grocery bags from the shopping cart to the trunk of your car.

3. ENCOURAGES SOCIALIZATION. Exercising with a medicine ball may help you make friends because so many ball exercises work best with two or more people. And since this type of training is especially effective for sports conditioning, teammates can train together.

4. ADDS VARIETY. Using a new piece of equipment does wonders for reviving a run-of-the-mill fitness program. Since medicine balls are so versatile, the exercises you can perform with them are limitless. And they're not just for elite athletes either. People of all fitness levels and ages benefit from this type of exercise.

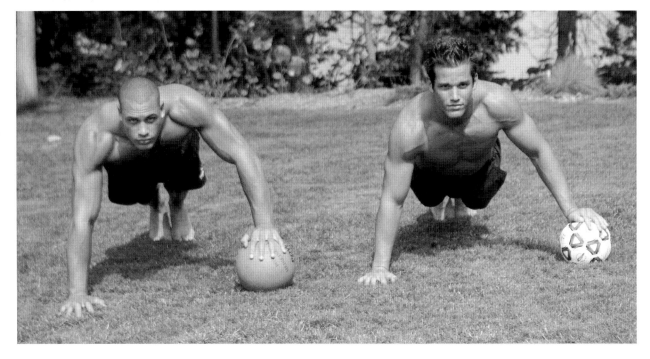

5. LETS YOU REVISIT YOUR YOUTH. In addition to the physical advantages of medicine-ball training, there is a psychological one: It can lift your spirits. Medicine balls have a playful quality, so they're enjoyable to use. Working with medicine balls makes you feel like a kid again.

PROGRAMMING—IN JUST THREE MOVES

ONE-HAND PUSH-UP. This is a classic push-up in the traditional form. Get down on the floor on your hands and knees. Place a medicine ball under one hand and position your other hand on the ground below you. Maintain the same hand position for this push-up, keeping your hands at shoulder width. The ball is going to create an unstable grounding for your hand. It will be difficult for you to balance the first few times you do this. Keep your body locked in a plank position the entire time without sagging in your midsection. Inhale as you lower your body to the ground, and exhale as you press. To intensify the exercise, you can switch the position of the ball to the other hand in the press-up. You have to use an explosive press and roll the ball over to the other hand, grasping the ball to stop it before you set the next push-up in motion.

THE CLEAN AND PRESS. This classic exercise is one of my personal favorites and will earn a place in your repertoire of exercises that deliver. The Clean and Press is an Olympic event, an exercise that uses every muscle in your body. Holding onto the medicine ball with both hands, lower the ball toward the ground by bending your knees and dropping your buttocks downward. Maintain a solid back so that your upper body does not bend too far forward. Your shoulders should be positioned above your hips. Lift the ball back up into the air with a full extension of both arms and repeat. The weight of the ball will provide enough resistance to get your heart rate up and challenge your muscles. This exercise can also be used as a form of aerobic movement for warming up.

The Clean and Press

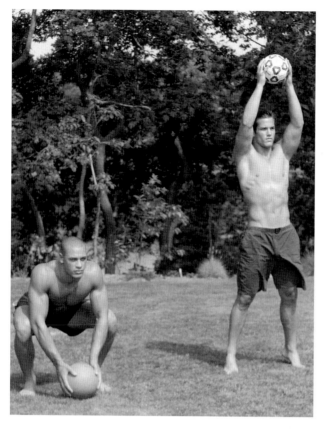

THE DYNAMIC LUNGE PRESS. This movement requires a partner to catch the ball after you toss it. The Dynamic Lunge Press incorporates a traditional lunge with a chest press for a compound exercise that requires power, balance, and deceleration skills. Starting and stopping the Dynamic Lunge Press will recruit different muscles than you have used in the past. Stand facing your partner, holding an appropriately weighted medicine ball at chest level. As you step forward into the lunge, toss the ball to your partner. Return to a standing position by pressing back with your foot and allow your partner to toss the ball back to you for the next go round. Repeat ten times per leg, allowing no rest.

The Dynamic Lunge Press

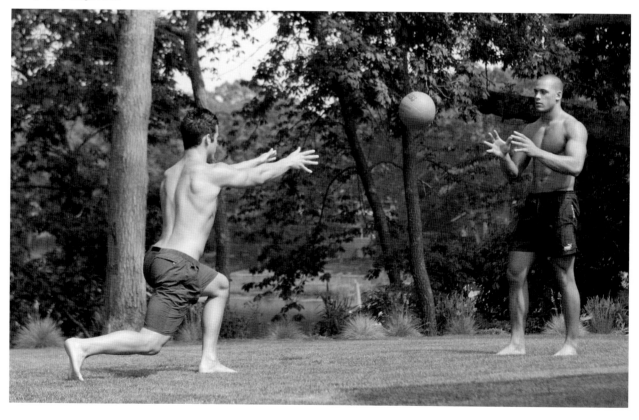

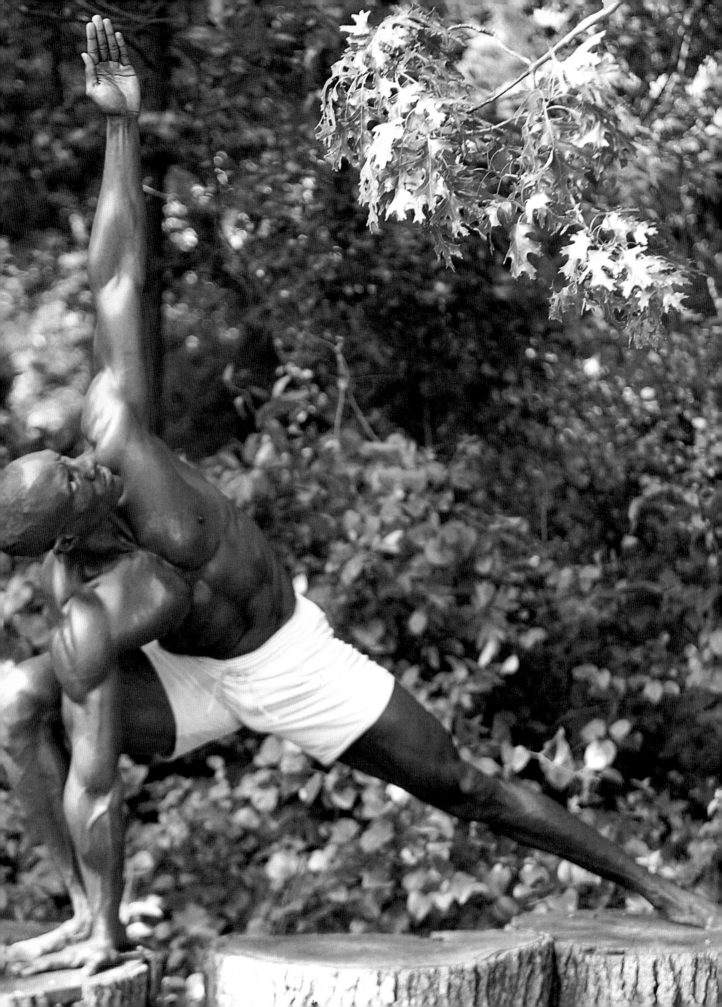

CHAPTER SIX

YOGA-INSPIRED TRAINING

WHAT IS IT?

Interest in yoga is surging throughout the world. This popular practice has roots in India, dating back at least thousands of years. Early references to yoga are found in the spiritual texts of the Vedas, Upanishads, and the Bhagavad-Gita. Pantanjali's yoga sutras (the Eightfold Path) are still widely studied and practiced today. The sutras form the basis of much of the modern yoga movement.

WHAT IS THE BENEFIT?

Yoga's numerous health benefits, its potential for personal and spiritual transformation, and its accessibility make it a practical choice for anyone seeking physical, psychological, and spiritual integration. The timeless applicability of yoga has helped bring it and other "alternative" models of healing into mainstream medicine. With increasing interest, media attention, and more people participating in yoga, it can be easy to get lost in the "yoga shuffle." Finding one's way through the ancient and modern yoga texts and institutions can be daunting. Unquestionably, the best way to understand yoga is to experience it. The following is a thumbprint sketch of a living tradition.

Yoga is a system of healing and self-transformation based on wholeness and unity. The word *yoga* itself means to "yoke"—to bring together. It aims to integrate the diverse processes with which we understand the world and ourselves. It touches the physical, psychological, spiritual, and mental realms we all inhabit. Yoga recognizes that without integration of body and mind, spiritual freedom and awareness—or what the yogis call "liberation"—cannot occur.

There is increasing evidence that yoga helps mental and emotional problems, such as anxiety and depression. Yoga promotes overall health and well-being, and can lead to increased ability to concentrate, greater capacity for creativity, richer relationships, enhanced sexuality, and enjoyment of life.

The aim of yoga (and the reason for the many different kinds of practices developed by the yogis) is to reach both a state of clarity and freedom from identification with the ups and downs of life and the fluctuation of thought. In ultimate terms, this means realizing one's true nature and achieving full self-knowledge. In a state of yoga (a unified state), the individual self is awakened to the connection with all of life—separation is revealed as an illusion. We are at one with the greater cosmic forces of nature, not divided from them. Yoga recognizes the divine nature of all beings and things. Yoga uses the term *enlightenment* to describe this state. Yoga's numerous health benefits make it a practical choice for anyone seeking physical, psychological, and spiritual integration.

CLEARING THE FOG

What does all this mean if you're new to the path of yoga? How does the physical practice of asana and breathing connect to the deeper meanings of yoga? The early yogis established the mind/body connection. Obstructions in both mind and body need to be cleared before peace of mind can unfold. The beginning yoga student need only start with the body and breath to sample the enhanced clarity and well-being that comes from a yoga practice. In addition to physical practices, there are other branches of the yoga tree that can equally lead to awareness and clarity.

HOW DO I GET STARTED?

BREATHING

In yoga, the energy of the body and mind is directly influenced by a force known as *prana*. *Prana* is the vital life energy that exists in different degrees everywhere in the universe. One purpose of hatha yoga is to increase this life force inside the body and mind, to enhance a person's well-being and energy, and eventually to lead one to higher states of meditation and clarity.

Breathing influences the mind and the emotions, and vice versa. Agitated breath can create an agitated mind, whereas a calm and focused breath can help us feel relaxed and at peace. *Prana* can also be influenced by the breath. In yoga, breathing techniques are used to increase *prana* (energy) and reduce obstructions in the body and mind. This practice is known as *pranayama*.

There are several different ways to breathe while practicing the asana (the positions or poses of most yoga practices). There are also many different breathing techniques in *pranayama*. *Caution:* If your breath feels strained, slow down or take a break. Breathing should never feel rushed or be painful. If you have allergies or asthma, you may need to modify the breath and/or consult your physician. It is always a good idea to find a knowledgeable teacher to help you with your breathing practice.

GENERAL BREATHING TIPS:

- Always inhale and exhale through your nose. This is the conscious cleansing yoga breath.

- Feel, listen, and visualize the breath moving in or out of your body.

- If you have allergies or sinus problems, try inhaling through the nose and exhaling through the mouth until the sinuses clear. If you are unable to breath through your nose, you can breathe through your mouth.

- Long, slow breathing is optimal.

- In the beginning, the exhale usually feels easier and longer than the inhale, and should be emphasized.

- Focus on the releasing quality of exhalation.

- Focus on the energizing quality of inhalation.

- Do not practice retention of breath if you have high blood pressure or are in the last trimester of pregnancy.

- Do not take in too much air at the beginning of your inhale. Let the breath enter and exit the body evenly.

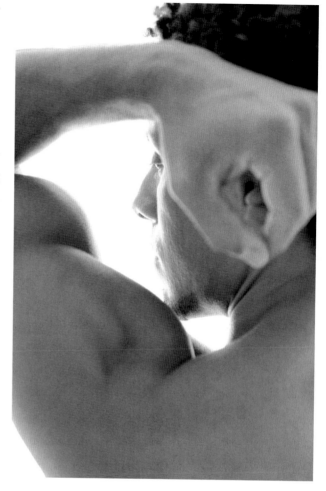

START BREATHING

Using the easy breath method, try this: Stand with arms at sides, feet together. Begin to inhale, raising your arms over your head while inhaling. Complete inhale. Pause. Begin to exhale, opening your arms to the side as you bend your torso forward as far as you comfortably can while exhaling. Complete the exhale. Pause. Feel free to bend your knees as you breathe. Repeat.

Apply this method to all of your yoga sequences and poses and your Pilates practice. If you move with the breath, your body will likely open and feel supported, and your mind will become more alert.

Each breath we take moves our spine through its primary movement patterns: extension and flexion. When our spine's movement is restricted, our breathing is restricted, and vice versa. If our workout ignores these restrictions, we stay in a rut of habitual patterns of restricted movement and breathing, limiting our capacity for grace, core stability, and emotional expression.

The natural way to invite full, deep breaths is to first develop a complete exhalation. Balls or cushions can be useful as aids to strengthen, open, and balance the structures that support a complete exhalation. These playful tools can help us to free up the pelvis, which is so deeply restricted by a lifetime of chair sitting.

When the iliopsoas (hip flexor) threading through the pelvis begins to lengthen and stabilize the link between legs and spine, we discover a deeper exhalation as our natural birthright. Once our exhalation is supported by an open, powerful lower body, our inhalation is free to fill and expand the chest. Our natural breathing rhythm can then do its healing work throughout our body and mind.

YOGA-INSPIRED ROUTINE

GENERAL RULES OF YOGA PRACTICE

Always use a sticky mat on all floor surfaces.

POSE (ASANA). Pay close attention to the detail of each position or pose. Use each description as a foundation for maximizing the benefits of the practice. Move into each pose slowly so that you minimize the risk of injury and become more aware of how you actually move through space. This awareness will also bring your mind into the body in ways you may have never experienced before.

HOLDING THE POSE. Go into the pose only as far as you are comfortable. The day I see a yoga competition is the day I stop being interested in health and wellness. Proper alignment is the most important component in any yoga pose. It is vital for you to practice each pose correctly and to recognize the sensation of the stretch and strength each position creates. If you are feeling any pain or discomfort at all stop and return to a comfortable position.

BREATHE AND RELAX. Always breathe naturally and through the nose. This will help you to breathe deeper, by using the midsection of your body to help push the air out of your lungs. Each pose can be held for as long as you wish, if you need a count to direct you, use five healthy breaths as a benchmark. Try to breathe deep into the lungs, and then relax completely between breaths.

FLOOR. It is important to have a nonskid floor for your practice. Our illustrations show a bare floor that is not slippery. Depending on the floor surface—carpet, wood, linoleum, and concrete—in your home, you can decide whether to purchase a sticky mat. They are widely used in yoga classes.

Always use a sticky mat on all floor surfaces.

YOGA-INSPIRED EXERCISES

SUN SALUTE. The Sun Salute can be used as an alternative warm-up to the Universal Warm-up used in

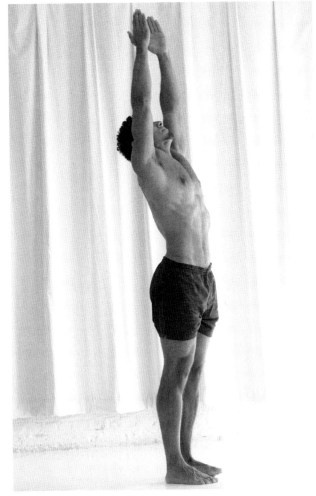

Hands Up

this book. The Sun Salute is a simple method that with time should become second nature to you. Think of it as a wake up to your body and your senses. The Sun Salute is not a series of poses that will be held for any length of time. The ritual is to move slowly and methodically, holding each pose for five seconds or so and then move into the next pose systematically. Try to develop a clean flow of movement from one position to the next.

Hands Up. From a standing position with your arms at your sides (neutral posture), brace your torso slightly and tighten your buttocks to ensure spine and pelvic stability. Bring both hands out to the sides of

Forward Bend

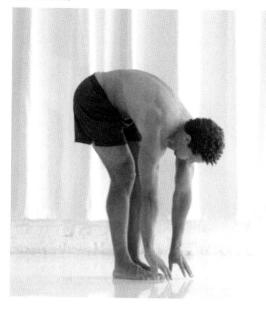

Lunge

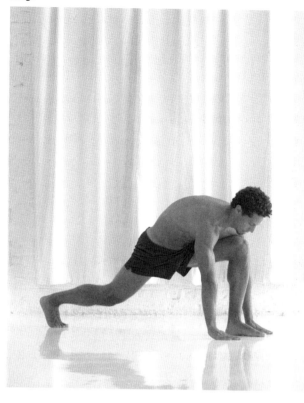

your body and raise them up into the air over your head with your palms facing each other. Reach onto the air and extend your body upward with your feet planted on the ground. Your upper and lower body should lean away from each other to stretch and open your midsection.

Forward Bend. Rotate your hands as you lower your arms down through the side pathway (not in front of your body), supporting your upper body with proper alignment of your spine to the floor. Your fingers can just touch the floor if you are flexible enough, or you can attempt to touch the floor and become aware that you need to focus special attention on the inflexibility of your hamstrings (back of the thigh). Keep your back long and your eyes looking down at your feet.

Lunge. With your fingers touching the floor and with a strong burst of power, jump one foot back behind you as far as you can comfortably. Your front foot should stay in place with your knee positioned directly

above the foot. Both hands can press down on the floor for added balance. Keep your attention on your midsection also, as you don't want to arch or round your back. Your head should maintain alignment with your spine. Make a mental note of the foot that is placed in front as you will have to change feet to keep the routine balanced. Change feet in succession while you are in the position.

Advamced Lunge

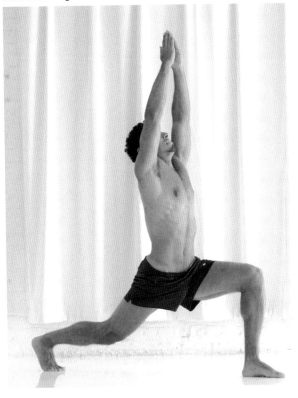

Push-up 2

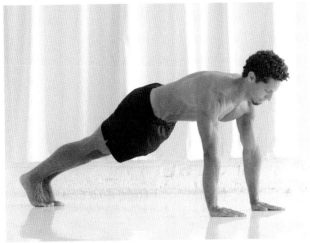

Push-up 1

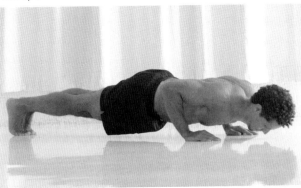

Advanced Lunge. To take the Lunge a step farther, use the last pose as a setup, and then simply raise your hands over your head as you did in the beginning of the Sun Salute. Extend your arms up enough to really feel your abs pull upward and stretch the front part of your hips.

Push-up. Bring both of your hands back down to the floor, directly below your shoulders. Both feet are now back behind you, and your body is positioned in a firm plank pose. This requires you to pull your navel up into your spine to support the middle of your body and maintain the extension of your head off your shoulders. Lower your body down to the floor with your elbows kept closer to your body than they would

be during a traditional push-up. The inside part of your upper arm could even slide against your side when you lower down toward the floor, stopping just before you touch it. Then press back up to a full plank position.

Up Dog. From the lower half of the push-up, drop your lower body down to the floor and allow it to rest going into this next position. The name of this pose leads you to the end of the pose. Press your arms, extending them to full length and raise your upper body toward the ceiling. This is similar to the Lunge where your torso lifts upward and stretches. Hold this extension and try to pull your shoulders down away from your ears, lengthening through your neck upward.

Up Dog

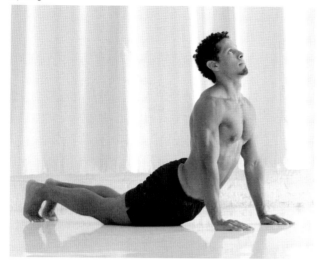

Downward Dog

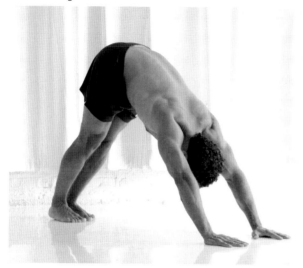

Downward Dog. Go right into this pose from the Up Dog pose. Hands maintain their position on the floor, but now you have to elevate through your hips upward through your coccyx. I mention this so that you have the advantage of lifting your buttocks and hips through the proper plane. When you get your hips up, your head should be positioned between your biceps. Your abs should be pulling your midsection up, and the stretch should be felt through the back of your legs. To intensify the stretch, drop your heels down toward the floor to lengthen your calves and the muscles that make up your ankles. Follow the same path back. Downward Dog, Up Dog, Push-up, Lunge, Advanced Lunge, Forward Bend, to Hands Up, then back to standing pose. Repeat the entire cycle as many times as you feel necessary. This alone is a workout

WARRIOR. Start this pose with your feet separated beyond shoulder width. Turn your attention to one side, looking ahead beyond your foot. Let's use the right side to start. While bending your right knee and positioning it over your right foot, turn your right foot,

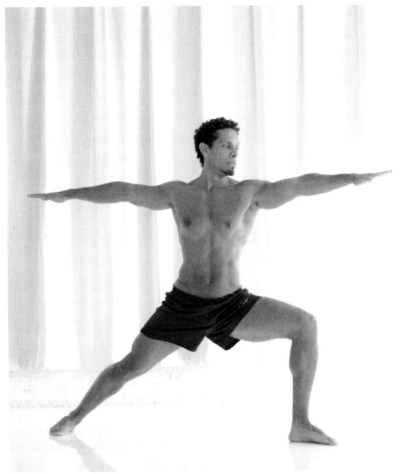

pointing directly away from the right side of your body. The other foot should remain in place so that your hip opens forward. Slowly elevate both arms directly out from the sides of your body, right arm over right leg and left arm over left leg. Your torso remains facing the same way it was when you started this pose, but your head will turn to look past your right hand. Your arms should stay positioned at shoulder level. Maintain the pose for a succession of five breaths and return to a standing pose. Repeat using the same progression on the left side.

Triangle 1

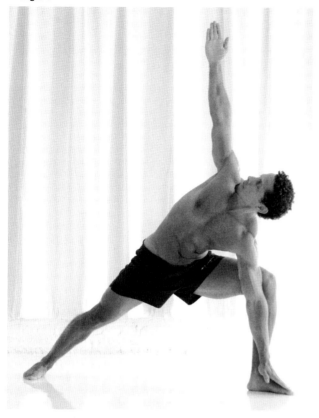

Triangle 2

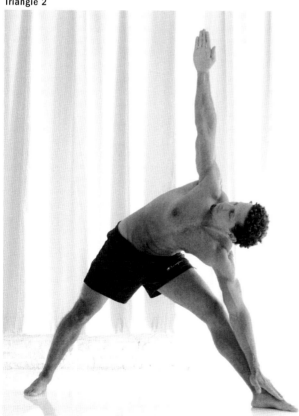

TRIANGLE. Start this pose with your feet separated wider than your shoulders. This pose is similar to the Warrior pose, only instead of bending at the knee, you will extend your right leg to shift your body weight evenly through both feet. Bring your upper body to the right from your chest and shoulders and bend from your waist to the right side. Bring your right hand down to the floor onto the top of your foot. You can modify this if you cannot reach your foot by bringing your hand to your shin or knee. Extend the left arm above your body at shoulder level and turn your focus beyond your left hand above you. Your head will turn to look up and therefore challenge the balance between front and back. Try to extend your bent knee, shifting your hips to the center. You'll feel a strength in your inner thigh. Maintain the pose for a succession of five breaths and return to a standing pose. Repeat using the same progression on the left side.

Tree 1

Tree 2

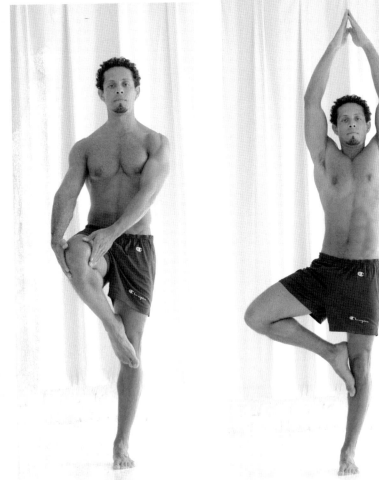

TREE. Start from a standing pose with both feet firmly planted on the ground. Keep your arms at your sides (neutral posture), maintaining a slight bracing of your torso and tightening of your buttocks to ensure spine and pelvic stability. Slide your right foot against the inside of your left shin, stopping at your knee. You can hold onto your right leg for security until you feel comfortable with the balance. This may even be as far as you can go. That is fine. Rotate your right knee out to the side of your body, keeping your right foot in place on your left leg. This will force you to reorganize your balance skill and requires your full attention. Bring both hands out to the sides of your body and raise them up into the air over your head with your palms facing each other. Reach into the air and extend your body upward with your feet planted on the ground. Your upper and lower body should extend away from each other to stretch and open your midsection. Maintain the pose for a succession of five breaths and return to a standing pose. Repeat using the same progression on the left side.

Reverse Right Angle

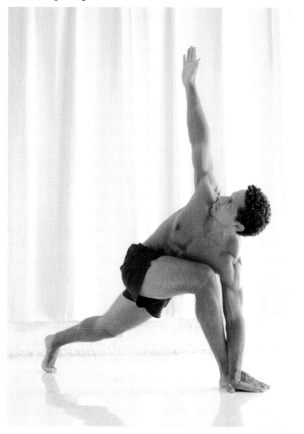

Reverse Right Angle II

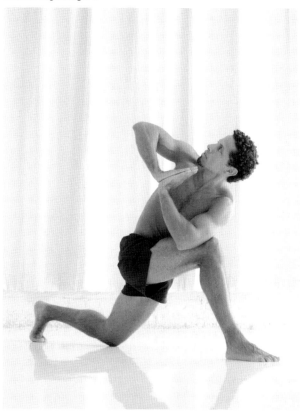

REVERSE RIGHT ANGLE. With your fingers touching the floor and with a strong burst of power, jump the left foot (as illustrated in the photo) back behind you as far as you comfortably can. Your right foot should stay in place with your knee positioned directly above the foot. Both hands can press down on the floor for added balance. Keep your attention on your midsection also. You don't want to arch or round your back. Your head should maintain its natural alignment. Position your left hand to the toe side of your right foot.

Reach your right arm into the air above your shoulder and look past your hand with your eyes. Keep your right knee in line with your right foot. Feel the rotation of your torso as you breathe into this pose. Bring your right arm back down to the floor and move your foot in to come out of the pose and repeat on the opposite side. This will take some practice because of the twist.

REVERSE RIGHT ANGLE II. From the Reverse Right Angle, you can advance the pose with your fingers touching the floor, and with a strong burst of power, jump your left foot (as illustrated in photo) back behind you as far as you comfortably can. Your right foot should stay in place with your knee positioned directly above your foot. Both hands can press down on the floor for added balance. Keep your attention on your midsection also, as you don't want to arch or round your back. Your head should maintain its natural alignment. Position your left hand to the toe side of your right foot. Reach your right arm into the air above your shoulder and look past your hand. Keep your right knee in line with your right foot. Feel the rotation of your torso as you breathe into this pose.

Advance the pose by bringing your left elbow to the outside of your right knee, reenforcing the twist in your torso. Bring your hands together and hold the pose for five breaths. Bring your right arm back down to the floor and move your foot in to come out of the pose. Repeat on the opposite side.

CHILD. Get down on the floor on your hands and knees. Sitting back on your feet with your coccyx down, allow your upper body to drape over your knees with your arms at your sides. You should feel the length of your spine here as you are supporting the rounded position of your back with your body. Let your head and neck relax and sit quietly for five breaths. Advance the level of this pose by lacing your

Child 1

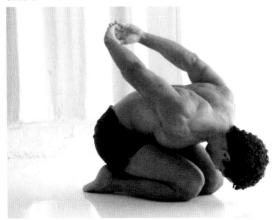

Bow 1

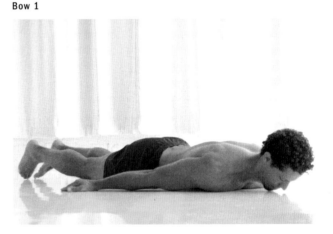

Child 2

Bow 2

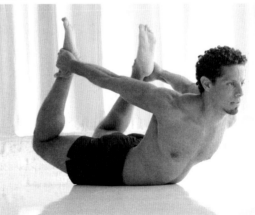

fingers together above your buttocks and slowly raising your hands into the air. If you feel any undue stress to your neck, relax this step in the pose. You will feel a stretch throughout your shoulders and chest. Hold for a count of five deep breaths and release.

BOW. Start this pose face down on the floor. You can rest your chin on the floor instead of pressing down on your nose. You should feel relaxed, with your arms and hands at your sides. Start with a gentle lift of the upper body as you bend your knees toward your buttocks. Keep your hips pressing into the floor as you try not to recruit the front of your leg for this pose. You will feel your hamstrings pull your feet up as you lift your upper body, reaching your hands to your feet. Grasp your feet with both hands and hold. Your shoulders will be elevated off the floor and your eyes should stay focused in front of you. You can add intensity to the pose by extending or pressing with the lower half of your leg. This will assist in lifting your upper body position off the floor. If this feels uncomfortable, release and lie back down on the floor. If not, hold for a count of five deep breaths and then release.

SITTING LEG EXTENSION. Turn over into a seated position with your legs extended in front of you. Sit tall on your coccyx and feel the stress in the backs of your legs as you begin to stretch. Move your hands to your sides and turn your fingers to the back. Feel your knee caps pulling back toward your upper body as you breathe. Extend downward through the arms, which will lift your chest and shoulders slightly higher, intensifying the tension behind your legs. It is vital to have an awareness of your spine in this pose; without knowing, you may have rounded your shoulders. Pay strict attention. Take five deep breaths for the pose and

Sitting Leg Extension

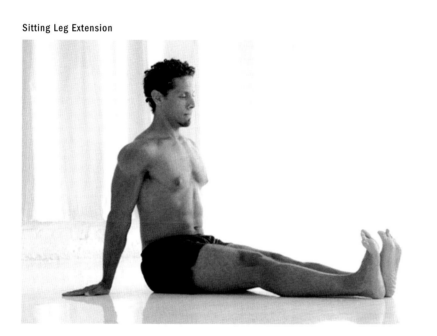

Sitting Wide-Leg Extension

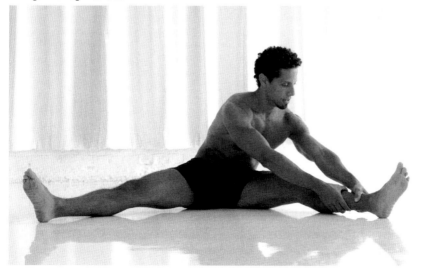

Rollback 1

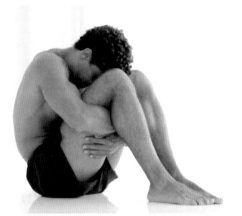

Hamstring Stretch

Rollback 2

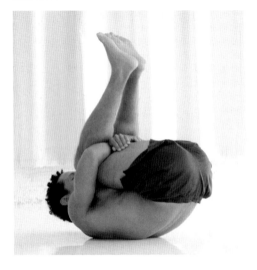

relax. Repeat the same effort on the other side and repeat the same number of breaths.

SITTING WIDE-LEG EXTENSION. Directly from the Sitting Leg Extension, separate your feet as wide as you feel comfortable. Maintain the best possible posture in the beginning to ensure you are squared out over your left leg first. Feel both sides of your coccyx on the floor. Draw your kneecaps back again as you did before in the Sitting Leg Extension, pressing through the heel of your left foot. Elevate your chest and tilt over your left leg while you extend your arms out to meet your hands to your ankle. Depending on your flexibility, you can go out as far as you wish, as long as you maintain

postural alignment. Take five breaths without bouncing forward and release. Repeat the same effort on the other side for the same number of breaths.

ROLLBACK. Come back to a seated position with your knees bent in front of you on the floor. Round your upper body over your knees and hold your legs with your arms. This will feel as though you are hugging yourself, and indeed you will be. Drop your head down to your knees and stay tucked back into this fetal position. With very little momentum, allow yourself to roll back and roll up again. Repeat this rolling a few times, but understand that your back is being massaged against the floor and that if you continue you may get dizzy or

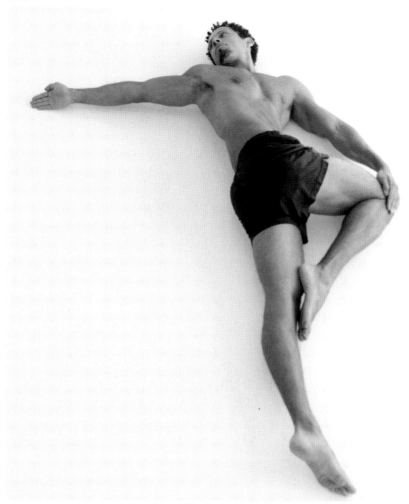

knee pointing to the ceiling. Lower your right leg to the left side of your left leg as far as you feel comfortable. Do not overstress this twist position; allow the stretch to take place as you breathe. By extending your right arm to the opposite side, you open your chest and shoulders and receive one of my favorite stretches and yoga poses. Take your time and do not rush this pose. Take five to six breaths and release by lifting up your right leg and coming back to full extension. Take the same path with your left leg and repeat for the allotted breaths.

QUESTIONS ABOUT YOGA

WHAT IF I'M NOT VERY FLEXIBLE?

The most common misconception that prevents people from trying yoga is that yoga is just stretching. Yoga is not solely about becoming flexible; instead the practice focuses on strengthening your body and spine in all directions. Yoga connects the body to the mind and keeps you in a serene state. Instead of fighting the thought of getting into the "head" that yoga requires for maximum benefits, give it a chance, feel the benefits, and your body will respond in ways you never expected.

light-headed. Stop after five or six times down on the floor and prepare for the next supine position pose.

HAMSTRING STRETCH. Lie on your back, trying to maintain a neutral body posture on the floor with shoulders relaxed and pulled down and away from your neck. Start by bending your right leg at the knee and drawing it into your midsection. With the help of your hands, hold your thigh in place as you lift your leg into a full exten-

sion above your hip. Do not pull on your leg; just assist the lengthening of the leg with both hands. You can intensify by straightening the other leg to the floor. Take five to six breaths as you allow your leg to receive the stretch and then release. Repeat on the left side.

TWIST. Start from the supine position on the floor by bending your right leg at the knee and drawing it into your center. Rest your right foot on your left knee with your

IS YOGA A CARDIOVASCULAR WORKOUT AND CAN I LOSE WEIGHT?

No matter what your level of fitness, you will find yoga very challenging. Each posture combines flexibility, strength, and balance to work your whole body from your bones to your skin. With persistence, patience, and dedication, you can lose inches and develop muscle tone and strength that might never be achieved with other forms of exercise. There are several forms of yoga to choose from. Use the yoga-inspired exercises in this book as a template for you to learn some of the language and positions. I want to inspire you to get to a yoga class. By using the routine here, you will be able to do that with confidence.

WHAT IS HOT YOGA?

There is a trend in the yoga universe called Bikram yoga. Bikram yoga is really hot—Literally. This yoga practice is a demanding twenty-six-pose (asana) series. A Bikram class is conducted in a heated room (around 100 plus degrees Fahrenheit) to warm up your whole body, allowing you to work deep into your muscles, tendons, and ligaments and change your body from the inside out. In yoga practices, the Sun Salute will help you warm your body naturally, but this takes time. The Bikram yoga philosophy suggests that the heat element helps your body warm up through the environment of the room, and therefore you get more work in a shorter period of time.

Bikram yoga, as well as many other forms of yoga, is a process that can reduce the symptoms of many chronic diseases, such as diabetes, pain, bulging disk/back pain, anorexia/bulimia, chronic fatigue, high cholesterol, and overweight, and is an excellent preventive activity for parts of the body that are healthy. The class is designed for all levels, first-time students and experienced practitioners alike. In time, you'll learn to focus your mind and control your breath, leading you to work harder, deeper, and calmer. As you improve with practice, you will realize the true meaning of yoga—a union of the body, mind, and spirit.

WHY THE HEATED ROOM?

The room is intentionally heated to warm your muscles and allow you to work deeper and safer. The heat also heals, helps prevent injuries, and promotes sweating, which flushes toxins from your body.

Bikram yoga is practiced in special schools and studios around the United States and is now finding its way around the world. You can find a studio near you via their official Web site. If you are considering another yoga class at your club or in a studio, there are some things that you should modify if you have any previous injuries and/or preexisting conditions.

Always tell the instructor this is your first time; check your ego at the door.

Keep your knees slightly bent to reduce the stress on your lower back.

Rest when you need to.

Do not compete with the others in the room; they may be more experienced.

Wear comfortable clothes.

Drink water throughout the session.

Try a basic or beginner class first to get you used to the format and practice.

CHAPTER SEVEN

PROGRAMMING STRATEGIES:

THE ROUTINES

PILATES-INSPIRED ROUTINE = ABS

FOR THE NOVICE

(Perform in order of exercises.)

Breathing Prep 8–10 Reps

Spinal Roll Up 10 Reps

The Hundred 10 × 10 Reps

Leg Circles 12 Reps each leg

THE MINIMALIST—TIME EFFICIENCY—FIVE MOVES

(Perform in order of exercises.)

Spinal Roll Up 10 Reps

The Hundred 10 × 10 Reps

Hip Lift with Twist 8–10 Reps

Leg Pull 8–10 Reps

Teaser 5–8 Reps

TOTAL BODY CONDITIONING—GOING BEYOND

(Perform in order of exercises.)

Breathing Prep—Ab Prep 8–10 Reps

Spinal Roll Up 10 Reps

The Hundred 10 × 10 Reps

Double Leg Stretch 8–10 Reps

Leg Circles 12 Reps each leg

Spinal Twist 5 Reps per side

Teaser 5–8 Reps

Side-Lying Side Leg Lift 5–8 Reps

Hip Lift with Twist 8–10 Reps

Leg Pull 8–10 Reps

Saw 5–8 Reps

EVERY TIME YOU TRAIN

Runners Stance—ten times per leg
(see page 68)

L-Shape Chest Stretch—ten times per arm
(see page 68)

Hip Flexor C-Curve Stretch—ten times per arm
(see page 69)

Lat Pull on the Ball—fifteen times (see page 70)

ON THE BALL ROUTINES =
STRENGTH

FOR THE NOVICE—BEGINNING WORKOUT

Incline and Flat Chest Press on Ball

Ball Seated Overhead Shoulder Press

Swimmer

Seated Ball Biceps Curl

On the Ball Triceps Extensions

Floor Bridge

Ball Tuck

Ball Crunch

SETS AND REPS: *Perform each exercise in order—two sets of eight to twelve repetitions.*
RHYTHM COUNT: *Three down, hold for two, two up.*

Hamstring Stretch

Side Stretch

THE MINIMALIST—TIME EFFICIENCY—FIVE MOVES (NO WEIGHTS)

Feet on Ball Push-up

Wall Squat

Single Leg Pull

Ball Tuck

Ball Roman Twist

SETS AND REPS: *Perform each exercise in order—two to three sets of twelve repetitions.*
RHYTHM COUNT: *Three down, hold for two, two up.*

Total Body

TOTAL BODY CONDITIONING—
GOING BEYOND—ADVANCED CYCLE

WORKOUT

Ball Wall Squat

Single Leg Floor Bridge

Dynamic Lunge Press

Ball Crunch

Ball Roman Twist

Unilateral Chest Press on Ball

Unilateral Ball Flye

Ball Pull Over

Ball Pikes

Ball Switch (upper to lower)

Ball Seated Forward Shoulder Raise

Ball Seated Lateral Raise

Ball Seated Overhead Shoulder Press

Upper Body Hyperextensions

Lower Body Hypers

Seated Ball Biceps Curl

On the Ball Triceps Extensions

SETS AND REPS: *Perform each cycle twice/twelve repetitions per exercise.*

RHYTHM COUNT: *Three down, hold for two, two up.*

Hamstring Stretch

Side Stretch

Total body

SPLITS
UPPER BODY ONLY

Unilateral Chest Press on Ball

Hands on Ball Push-up

Unilateral Ball Flye

Ball Pull Over

Ball Hyperextensions

Ball Seated Lateral Raise

Ball Seated Overhead Shoulder Press

Ball Preacher Curl

Seated Ball Biceps Curl

On the Ball Triceps Extensions

Ball Dips

SETS AND REPS: *Perform each exercise in order—two to three sets of twelve repetitions.*

RHYTHM COUNT: *Three down, hold for two, two up.*

LOWER BODY ONLY

Ball Wall Squat

Floor Bridge

Floor Bridge Hip Rotations

Single Leg Floor Bridge

Single Leg Pull

Additional exercises described only

Lateral Lunge

Walking Lunge

Step-ups

SETS AND REPS: *Perform each exercise in order—three sets of twelve repetitions.*

RHYTHM COUNT: *Three down, hold for two, two up.*

CORE ONLY

Ball Crunch

Ball Roman Twist

Ball Switch (upper to lower)

Swimmer

Upper Body Hyperextensions

Lower Body Hypers

Ball Tuck

Ball Pike

SETS AND REPS: *Perform each exercise in order—two to three sets of twelve repetitions.*

RHYTHM COUNT: *Three down, hold for two, two up.*

YOGA-INSPIRED ROUTINE = FLEXIBILITY

FOR THE NOVICE

Sun Salute

    Hands Up

    Forward Bend

    Lunge

    Push-up

    Up Dog

    Downward Dog: retrace the steps back to complete cycle

Three Full cycles of the Sun Salute.

THE MINIMALIST—TIME EFFICIENCY— FIVE MOVES

    Warrior

    Downward Dog

    Reverse Right Angle

    Triangle

Twist

Perform each pose in order twice—holding each pose for five breaths.

TOTAL BODY CONDITIONING—GOING BEYOND

Sun Salute

    Hands Up

    Forward Bend

    Lunge

    Push-up

    Up Dog

    Downward Dog: retrace the steps back to complete the cycle

Warrior

Triangle

Tree

Reverse Right Angle

Reverse Right Angle II

Sitting Leg Extension

Child

Bow

Rollback

Hamstring Stretch

Twist

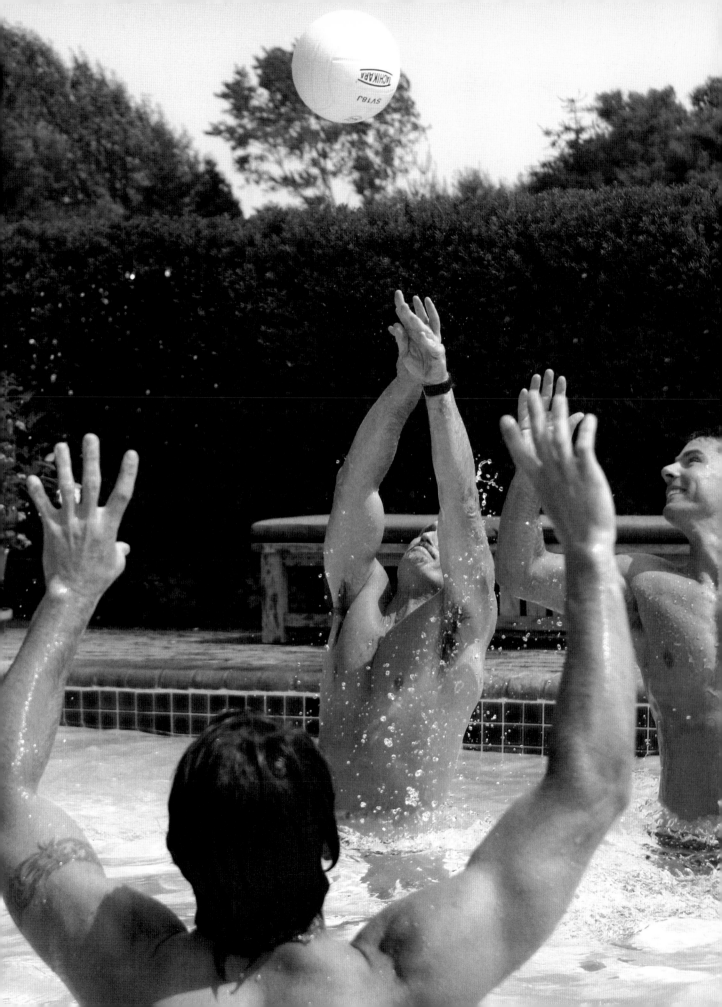

THINK BEFORE BUYING HOME
EXERCISE EQUIPMENT

With *Beyond Basic Training* and the programming strategies I have introduced you to, I want to keep the list of items you're required to buy to a minimum. You can set up for training at home for seventy-five dollars or less. The routines and exercises in this book require the following tools. A list of places to get these items is in the resource guide at the end of this book.

A stability ball (55-65 cm most commonly used)

A sticky mat

Hand weights

Water

A medicine ball (3-6 kg)

If you want to have more equipment than the above listing, consider the following:

If you are going to buy a piece of exercise equipment—either cardio or strength equipment—for your home, do not buy a unit that has every bell and whistle. All that stuff looks good, but you don't need half of those fancy features. Think about what you really need and want. Sometimes monitoring every cell of your body is not necessary for a good workout. Often gadgets and accessories go underused and misunderstood. The most important informational or support feature to get when buying home cardio equipment is an accurate heart-rate monitor. When it comes to strength-training equipment, get something that is easily adjustable and is appropriate for the space you have available. You want this to be a positive invest-

ment, and you need enough room around the unit to maneuver.

With so many new and improved machines, sometimes the essentials get left behind. Look for quality construction and durable surfaces. There is nothing worse than getting a piece of exercise equipment that you bought one late night from a shopping channel, then when you unpack the treadmill or abdominal machine it is nothing like the one they described.

Test drive: Would you buy shoes without trying them on? Get on the bike and ride for twenty minutes, get on the treadmill and find out how it works before you consider it. Try pushing and pulling all the weight positions as well to see if the machine meets your need and goals. You don't have to make the buying of a piece of equipment the cheap way of getting in a good workout, but you should know how it feels and how it sounds before you bring it home.

Look at the range of manufacturers. Go to a store that sells a wide variety of equipment, or visit a Web site to get as much information as you can before you choose the right unit for you. That way you can also see and feel the difference between manufacturers. The difference will not only be in price, but also in design.

Something that looks good in an infomercial may not be right for you. Keep it simple. If you have a hard time with coordination, consider sticking with a machine that you know you can succeed with. I have seen as many of these gimmicks as you have, and I have been on the side of the manufacturer as well. Demonstrations have to make a machine look as though it were as easy as sliding down a hill. One button, one pin, one strap. It's never that easy. Go for something tried and true and that you will use.

Make sure that the unit you purchase has a safety

record. Does the treadmill have a turn-off switch or railings for your hands should you become dizzy? Does the Total Gym adjust to your height and weight? Will that bike hurt my back?

Ask questions before you buy. It is important for you to talk not just to someone from the manufacturers, but to some owners. They will tell you the truth. They will sing the machine's praises if they have found success and tell you so. Go to your friends as well. They will be more likely to give you an honest answer and a strong recommendation if the machine deserves one.

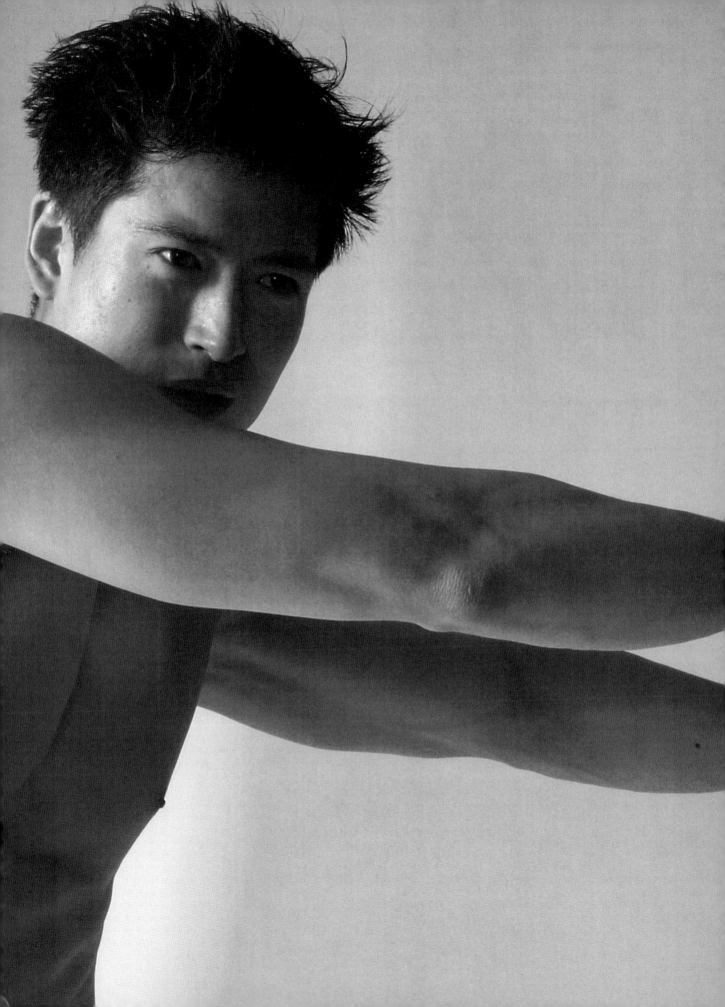

PART III

INTEGRATION

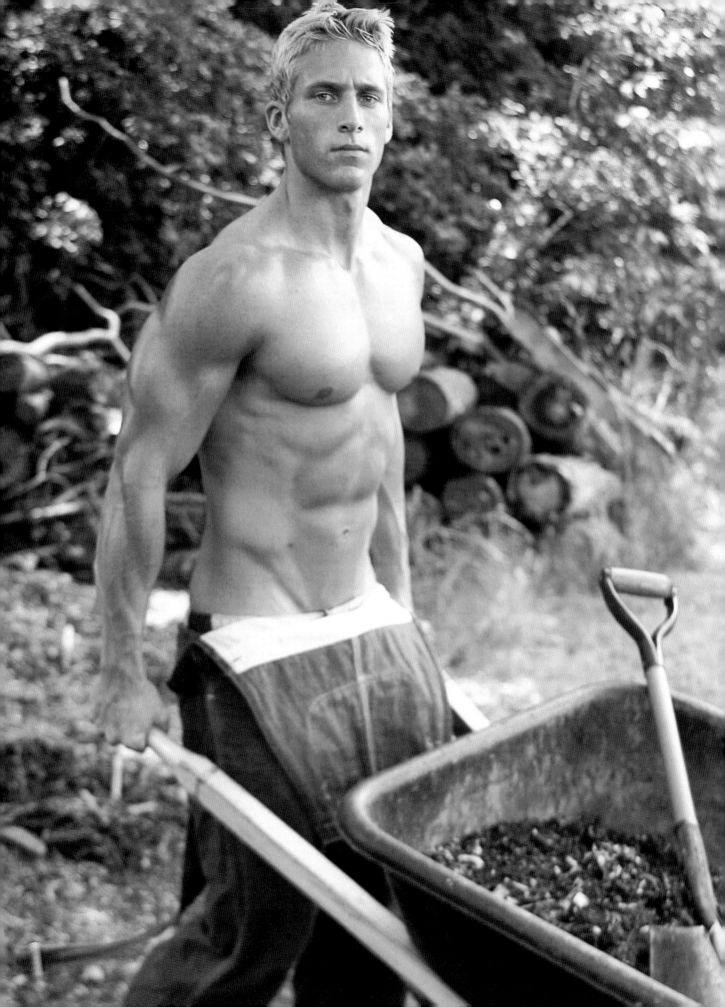

CHAPTER EIGHT

CROSSTRAINING

WORK VERSUS PLAY

Have you ever seen a fat runner? I never have. Have you ever seen a fat exercizer? I see them every day. More people perform aerobic exercise than any other fitness activity, yet many of them remain, at various levels, basically unfit. Why is this and what can be done about it?

AEROBICS IS NECESSARY AND AVAILABLE

Aerobic exercise takes many forms. First, you have walking, followed by jogging, then running. To get off your feet, you can ride a bike, tug on a rowing machine, or jump onto a stair climber or elliptical rider you see advertized on TV. Whatever the activity is, if you continue it long enough, you'll obtain aerobic conditioning. Remember that exercise should be enjoyable and refreshing. Forget that old "No Pain, No Gain" mentality; it's simply not true for the life-extension enthusiast. Start any aerobic exercise at a pace that's comfortable with your physical condition, then gradually accelerate the tempo and frequency of your workouts as you adapt to your new lifestyle. In a short time, you'll recognize numerous health benefits.

WHAT IS AEROBIC EXERCISE? BACK TO BASICS

Depending on the activity or task at hand, the body innately selects one of two basic energy sources as fuel. For powerful and explosive tasks that are interrupted with rest intervals—like weight lifting, football, etc.—the body will choose carbohydrates as the dominant fuel source. This is called "anaerobic metabolism." For long, sustained, uninterrupted activities, performed at submaximal efforts—like jogging or swimming—the body will utilize oxygen and fat as fuel sources. This is referred to as "aerobic metabolism." Sustained activities are better fueled with fat and oxygen as these two energy sources are the most dense and abundant fuels—the body never has to worry about running out. In contrast, running out of carbohydrate fuel (in the form of glucose or glycogen) can happen within seconds of an intense power burst.

The analogy I use when teaching the body's energy system is that of a rocket ship. Rockets are launched into outer space with several power, or fuel, boosters. The first booster is used to explode the rocket—and its massive weight—up off the ground. Once that booster is depleted of fuel, it disengages and the second booster propels the rocket even farther into the sky. Once the final booster is reached, the rocket is dependent on a fuel source that will carry it throughout the rest of its mission, which is of long duration in comparison to take-off. During exercise, your body acts like a rocket ship. When activity begins, your body relies on immediate and fast-burning fuel sources—carbohydrates. If you repeat an explosive burst after taking a replenishing rest, the body will again select carbohydrates as fuel. However, when activity persists for a long duration and is less intense, such as that in most aerobic workouts, carbohydrate stores deplete and/or are bypassed early in the routine, and the body automatically shifts to a fuel mixture of oxygen and fat in the wake of carbohydrate depletion.

INTENSITY

Generally speaking, the duration of aerobic exercise should extend no less than twenty minutes, with sessions exceeding thirty to forty-five minutes being ideal. During exercise, the cardiorespiratory systems are forced to function above a resting level and at submaximal levels; this is referred to as the "aerobic threshold" or "aerobic range." Experts say that 60 to 85 percent of maximum heart rate (MHR) is the range where best aerobic benefits are obtained—you'll see why later.

MAXIMIZING RESULTS

1. Scientific data indicates that the amount of energy expended *after* an aerobic workout tends to be very small.

2. The number of calories burned during recovery is dependent upon the intensity of the workout.

3. Conventional aerobic exercise is effective at burning body fat only during the activity itself.

For those needing to lose excess body fat, and only able to use aerobics to accomplish this objective, training frequency must increase. Let's look at the real differences between the sprinter and the aerobicizer.

A sprinter's training and competition requires a series of explosive performances—the hundred-meter dash, for instance, is less than ten seconds, and these athletes are lean, muscular, and healthy. In training, a sprinter will perform a sprint drill, rest, perform another sprint drill, followed by another rest period, and repeat that cycle until the work-out requirements have been fulfilled for the day. In comparison, an aerobic athlete may train for the same time period as the sprinter (or anaerobic athlete) but aerobic workouts are continuous, with no rest intervals.

If aerobicizers train nonstop throughout the entire duration of their workouts, burning calories without hesitation, why do so many of them have difficulty retaining lean muscle tissue and keeping fat storage under control? Conventional aerobics do not stress the muscular system; primary stress is to the heart and lungs. Energy is used (or burned up) to perform the workout but little is needed in postrecovery, as the body is not traumatized the way it is in anaerobic exercise.

Anaerobic activities emphasize the muscular system to a high degree. Intensity percentages begin at 75 percent and escalate to 100 percent. The bulk of true anaerobic training lies between 75 to 90 percent of maximum ability; this is called "the anaerobic range." Anaerobic training utilizes carbohydrates as fuel, mostly ignoring oxygen and fat during the workout itself. During anaerobic training, microtraumas are experienced to the muscles as anaerobic—or explosive—movements tear tissue on a microscopic level. The body's own defense mechanism for these types of injuries repairs the damage and rebuilds and strengthens the lean tissue of the body. Here's the amazing secret: postworkout repa-

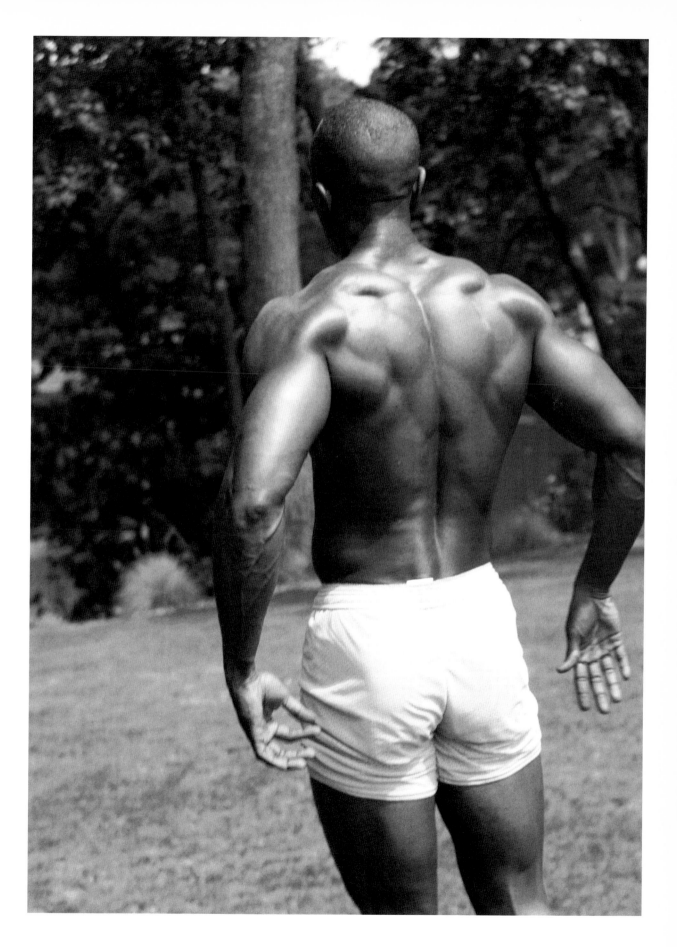

ration of damaged tissues that have been inflicted by anaerobics stimulates metabolism for several days after each workout and utilizes many energy sources, including fat, to fuel tissue remodeling. This is why the sprinter has an easier time staying leaner than his aerobic cousin. Also, lean tissue is metabolically active, meaning it burns more calories, even at rest. So those who strive to attain a higher degree of quality lean tissue will have an easier time keeping fat stores low.

To get the best of both worlds—aerobic conditioning for your heart and lungs, and anaerobic development of quality lean tissue—I suggest that many of your aerobic sessions be conducted with interval intensities. For instance, if you are walking, begin your workout at a comfortable pace, after you feel warmed up, speed up to a power walk or even a slow jog or run until you have difficulty breathing. Maintain that accelerated pace until you've had enough, then decelerate back to a pace you can endure comfortably. Continue this interval training throughout your workout. In essence, you'll be moving in and out of both the aerobic and anaerobic ranges all within the same workout.

The thing to understand about conventional aerobics is that on the days you're doing your aerobics, you're benefiting; but on the days you're resting, not much is being accomplished. This is why so many overload the frequency of their aerobic workouts. Ideally, I believe as is now the newer set standard by ASCM, no more than five aerobic workouts should be conducted each week; any more is excessive. Each workout might fluctuate between 30 to 60 minutes with occasional 90 to 120-minute sessions; like afternoon walks or bike rides. Overtraining sets in when one tries to rely on aerobics for total body conditioning. At first, overloading the body with this volume of training might seem to be manageable, but if the body is not completely recovered before your next workout,

your recuperative needs will compound themselves over time, and your results will stagnate or even regress. This is when you know you're overtraining.

If you try interval aerobics, on the days you're exercising, you'll benefit, and on the days you're resting, you're still receiving results! Interval aerobics will condition the heart and lungs and at the same time create the muscular trauma needed to ignite your postworkout metabolism and build the lean tissue you need. Isn't that amazing? It's like making a great investment and enjoying the interest. Plus, you don't have to exercise either as frequently or as long.

Interval aerobics can be applied to walking, biking, running, stair climbing, rowing, and all other forms of aerobic activity. You can also try alternating uphill and flat land while walking, biking, or running. Some of the new aerobic machines even have preset computer-interval courses that make interval aerobics easy to apply indoors.

GETTING BACK TO THE "WHY'S" OF AEROBICS

Aerobic exercise produces benefits you simply cannot live without. Getting a regular dose of aerobic exercise contributes to vibrant health and can extend mean life span. It benefits:

THE BRAIN

As with any activity, voluntary or involuntary, the brain is the master controller of the human body. Those who are sedentary don't spend enough time thinking about or doing things for their bodies. They also don't engage in physically challenging activities that require specialized skills to perform.

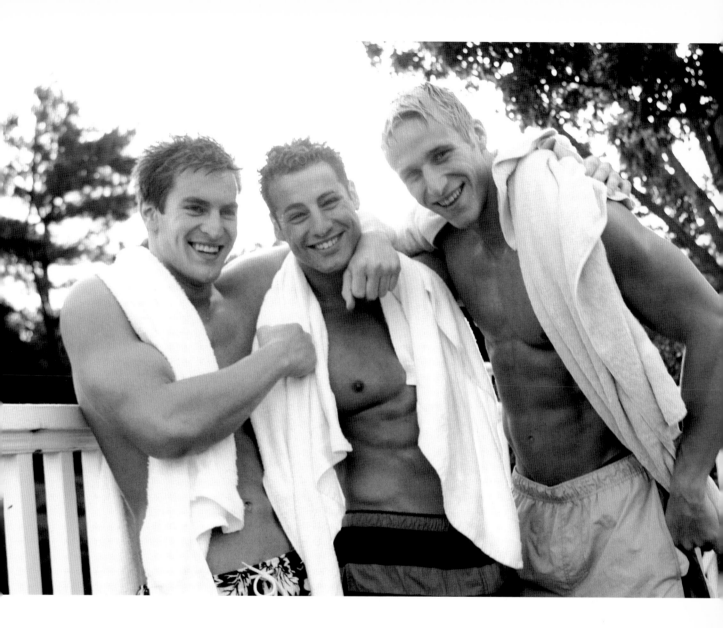

On the other hand, those who engage in exercise regularly are like pilots in the cockpit behind the controls of a sophisticated machine. Exercise requires billions of physiological actions that only the brain can pilot. As we condition ourselves, we have the ability to communicate with the various systems of our bodies and, in many ways, control our health. Once a satisfactory level of conditioning is achieved, the body and its various systems begin to operate in efficient harmony, largely due to improved brain function.

THE HEART

Conditioning the heart is probably the number-one reason why most people commit to aerobics, and aerobic exercise indeed targets the heart and its vascular system. The heart is a pump that, with each contraction, forces the circulation of blood throughout the body. With each heartbeat our cells receive the nourishment needed to survive as oxygen and other vital nutrients are pumped into these sites through our vascular system. The heart is a muscle, and the stronger your heart is the more easily it can circulate the blood we need to live. Inside the human body are approximately sixty thousand miles of blood vessels that act as pathways to oxygenate the body's tissues and unburden them of waste. If the heart is weak, it has to work overtime to accomplish these tasks, whereas a conditioned heart can force more blood throughout the body.

At rest, strong hearts don't need to beat as fast due to the fact that each beat is more forceful, whereas the weaker heart needs to pump more quickly and more often to maintain adequate blood flow, one reason for elevated blood pressure.

A normal heart rate is about 72 beats per minute (bpm). For those who exercise, the rate can reduce to below 60 bpm; (I've measured 48–54 bpm in a few of my students). If you're doing the math, that means a well-conditioned person can save a minimum of 12 heart beats each minute, 720 beats each hour, 17,280 beats each day, 518,400 beats each month, and 6,307,200 beats each year.

You don't have to be a mathematician to figure out that if you save over 6 million heart beats each year, you're bound to prevent the normal wear and tear that plagues so many people in our aging population. Try flexing your biceps 6 million times and see how that muscle feels.

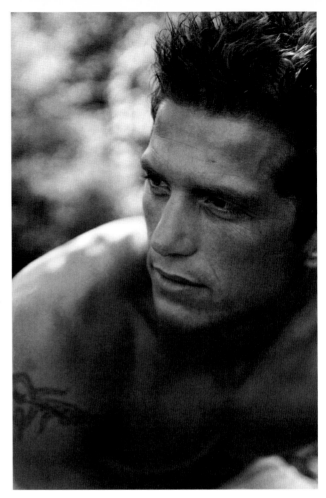

speeds, throughout the body, not only carrying the nutrients and oxygen we need to survive, but also removing toxins at the same time.

VASCULAR CLEANSING

As heart rate accelerates during exercise, internal cleansing is also taking place. The simplest analogy is that of a house's plumbing system. When water is forced to flow through the plumbing on a regular basis—such as running faucets—the inner linings of those tubal pathways remain relatively clean. As the water surges through the pipes on a regular basis, waste materials are more easily eliminated. The same holds true for the human body. With each aerobic workout, accelerated heart rate forces more blood, at faster

THE RESPIRATORY SYSTEM

Another target system emphasized during aerobic exercise is your respiratory system, the system that allows you to inhale air, absorb vital oxygen, and exhale toxic gases like carbon dioxide. The lungs are the primary organs of the respiratory system. The lining of your two lungs are made up of spongy tissue that contains millions of tiny holes called alveoli. The alveoli enlarge as we inhale, and the lungs expand. As we exhale, the alveoli shrink and the lungs constrict.

With each inhalation, oxygen is taken into the body and penetrates the lungs, eventually seeping into the circulatory system. The lungs are responsible for supplying the bloodstream with oxygen, which is then transported to the tissues via the circulatory system. Human life is dependent on oxygen. Going without oxygen for just a few minutes ends a life. And even though we might receive just enough oxygen to allow us to function on a day-to-day basis, being deprived of adequate supplies inevitably guarantees a road that's filled with maladies.

It's wise to condition the system that provides the most vital element of life. With literally thousands of deep breaths accumulating during each aerobic session, the lungs and the respiratory system strengthen, attaining an enhanced ability to supply an abundance of oxygen to all body cells. Even at rest, the well-conditioned respiratory system will provide greater oxygenation. Those who engage in regular aerobic training will feel fresher, clearheaded, and more cognitive no matter what they're doing.

Headaches, memory loss, fatigue, and lack of concentration are just a few conditions aerobic exercise can alleviate (and even cure).

THE MUSCLES

Muscles are basically composed of two fiber types: (1) Fast-twitch muscle fibers (FT), and (2) slow-twitch muscle fibers (ST). The FT fibers are used for short bursts of energy, are very powerful, require carbohydrates as fuel, and fatigue very easily. ST fibers are used for sustained activity, are weak in comparison to the FT fibers, utilize oxygen and fat as fuel, and are resistant to fatigue. If I told you to walk a hundred meters, at the end of that walk you'd be breathing relatively easily, would be able to carry on a conversation, and could continue walking indefinitely. On the other hand, if I told you to perform an all-out sprint for the same distance, by the time you crossed the finish line you'd be gasping for air and would need a lot of time to rest before proceeding with any other activity. The body uses two very different and distinct systems to carry out each task.

Training and developing both the FT and ST muscle fibers is the ideal protocol for optimum health, appearance, and performance. As we age, we naturally use fewer of the FT fibers. Consequently, these fibers atrophy. Strength, energy, and the ability to perform quick movements tends to diminish with each passing year. The concept of interval aerobics works perfectly well for enhancing the integrity of both the ST and FT muscle fibers. I'm convinced that this methodology will contribute greatly to developing leaner physiques of impressive muscular tone and symmetry with more stamina and better overall health.

TARGET HEART RANGE: ATTAINING AND MAINTAINING THE AEROBIC THRESHOLD

As previously discussed, according to many fitness experts, the target intensity range to perform aerobic activity lies between 60 and 85 percent. This is the rate at which the heart is beating during exercise and which is calculated from your maximum heart rate (MHR). We know that at rest our hearts should beat between sixty to seventy-two times each minute. Once we begin to exercise, that rate increases. When the heart attains a beating pace between 60 and 85 percent of its MHR (see formula), studies suggest that this is the intensity, or pace, that should be sustained until that work-out time expires.

My method of interval aerobics moves your heart

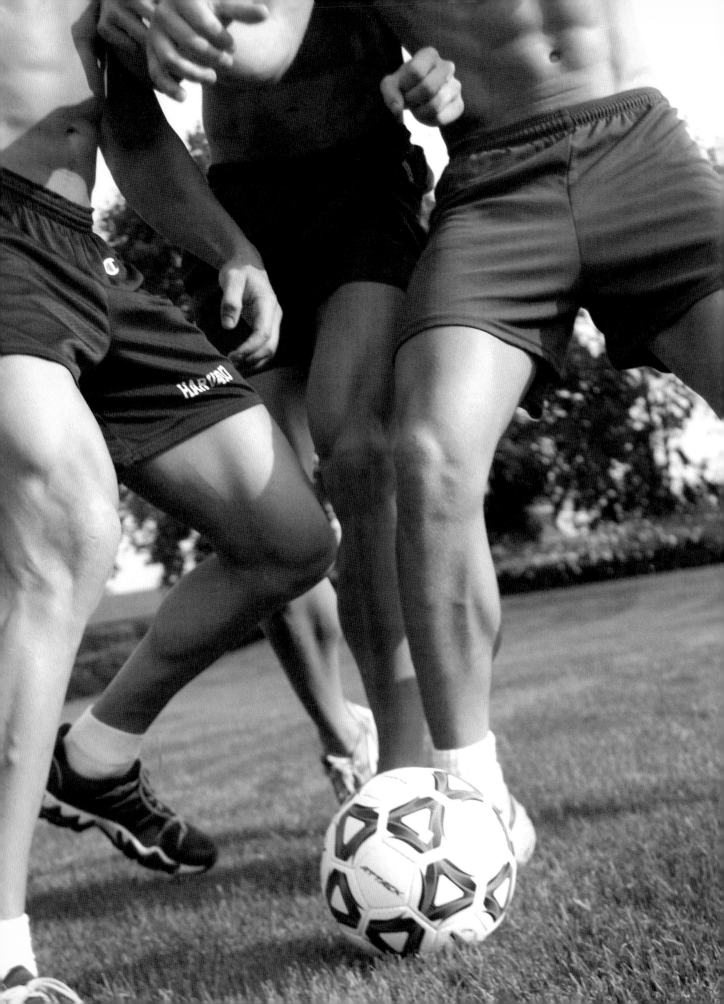

rate in and out of the conventional range of 60 to 85 percent. With interval aerobics, you'll avoid a one-sided energy source and burn carbohydrates, oxygen, and fat. You'll also train both the anaerobic and aerobic systems of the body and condition the heart and lungs and muscles.

If you calculate the fluctuations of your heart-rate throughout an interval aerobic session, you'll discover that your average heart-rate, or overall intensity, measures well within the range needed to provide excellent results.

To determine your heart-rate percentages follow this formula:

1. 220 MINUS YOUR AGE EQUALS YOUR MAXIMUM HEART RATE (MHR) OR HEART BEATS PER MINUTE (BPM).

2. MULTIPLY MHR BY 60 PERCENT, THEN BY 85 PERCENT; THIS IS YOUR AEROBIC RANGE AND THE INTENSITY YOU SHOULD REACH FOR THE DURATION OF THE AEROBIC TIME PERIOD.

Here's an example for an individual fifty years of age; (figures are rounded):

220 – 50 (AGE) = 170 (MAXIMUM HEART RATE)

170 × 60 PERCENT = 102 (BEATS PER MINUTE) (MODERATE AEROBIC INTENSITY)

170 × 85 PERCENT = 144 (BEATS PER MINUTE) (HIGH AEROBIC INTENSITY)

As long as this fifty-year-old aerobic participant performs his/her workouts, maintaining a heart rate (or average BPM) between 102 to 144, results are guaranteed. Interval aerobics may increase BPM above 85 percent and plummet BPM below 60 percent during the bursts of power and relaxation phases, respectably. Don't worry, your training heart rate will average out, and you'll attain aerobic conditioning.

ACTIVITY SELECTION LIST

HIGH IMPACT	LOW IMPACT
Jogging	Walking
Running	Biking
Aerobic dancing	Cross-country skiing
Basketball	Skating/blading
Swimming*	Swimming
Step class	Rowing
Rope jumping	Stair Climbing

GENERAL GUIDELINES

To begin an aerobic program, I suggest the usual checkup from your physician to obtain the "green light" to proceed. After that, it's wise to make a selection of the activities you'll perform, then set your schedule—both days and specific times.

I suggest a frequency of three to five aerobic workouts each week. If you're a beginner, start with ten to fifteen-minute workouts three times a week, then add five minutes every other workout until you reach thirty

*Swimming may impose high-impact shock to the shoulder apparatus. (*NOTE:* High-impact and low-impact aerobics refers to the shock, or pounding, experienced during the activity.)

minutes; you can go as high as sixty minutes. If you're going to try interval aerobics, I suggest that you first endure a conventional aerobic program for at least a month to condition yourself. At the same time, you should include some weight training, which isolates the FT fibers of the muscles you'll stress most with your activity. For instance, if you walk, jog, or run, it's wise to strength-train the knees, ankles, and lower back. If you swim, cross-country ski, or use a rowing machine, perform some upper body resistance exercises to strengthen and prepare the upper body muscles.

During your interval aerobic workout session, I suggest shorter durations as compared to a conventional session. A time reduction of 25 percent is average. For example, if you're normally performing sixty-minute aerobic workouts, reduce your time to forty-five minutes with the intervals. Cutting your work-out time with interval aerobics should in no way make you feel guilty. Interval aerobics burns more calories during a shorter period of time than conventional aerobics; plus, you'll burn more calories even at rest. If you use good judgment and listen to your body, you shouldn't have problems with overtraining and should experience year-round progress. Aerobics are terrific, but my little twist with the inclusion of intervals will help you achieve better results faster.

TRAINING TO RUN YOUR FIRST 5K

So you've started a walking program and, after a few weeks of consistent improvement, you feel you're ready to pick up the pace and run your first 5k race. Whether your goal is personal fitness, a sense of community, or a pure sense of accomplishment, you can find yourself at the finish line on race day.

A 5k race is the perfect length to aim for as a beginner. Begin by setting attainable goals to keep you motivated and give yourself ample time to move to the next level. If you train correctly and follow a good eight-to ten-week training program, running can lead to a lifetime of fitness.

SET ATTAINABLE GOALS

The length of a 5k is a relatively easy goal to reach as a novice runner, but it may also challenge the expert runner depending on intensity and speed. Start out with a simple program that allows you to succeed and move forward only when you feel comfortable with your current stage. To avoid burnout or injury, do not push your limits. Remember that your main goal is to reach the finish line. For your first race you should plan on enjoying the run and feeling good for having completed your goal.

IMPROVE YOUR HEART AND HEAD

Accomplishing your goal improves your self-esteem and keeps your cardiovascular system in tune. A regular training program includes exercising for at least thirty minutes three to five times per week, which falls within basic cardiovascular fitness guidelines. Running can lead to a feeling of freedom and independence, and it is also one of the best ways to alleviate stress since it releases alpha waves in your brain, leaving you relaxed and invigorated.

TAKE YOUR TIME

Depending on your training base, an eight- to ten-week program should be just enough time to have you running for the full thirty minutes, which is the ap-

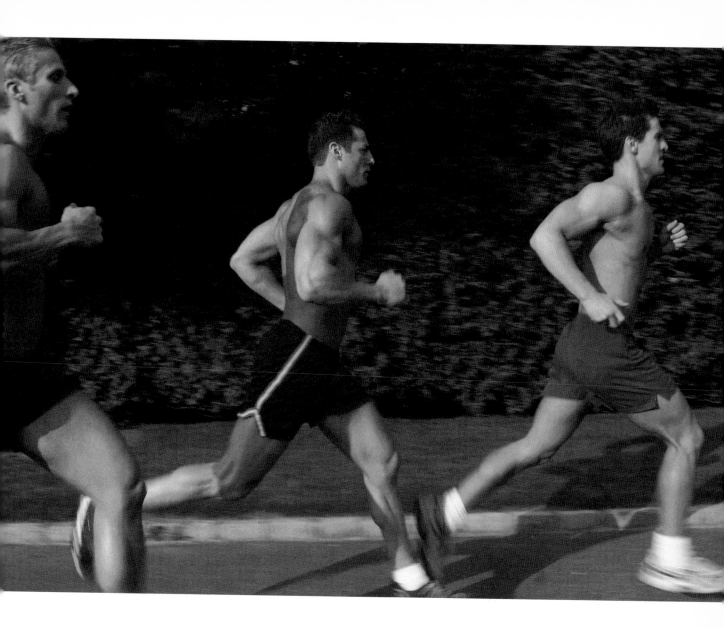

proximate time it will take you to complete your first 5k. Your first step should be a complete medical exam to make sure it is safe for you to begin a running program. Begin with a walk/run program four times per week for twenty to thirty minutes.

If you have not previously been involved in a walking program, it may be best to start with an eight-day walking routine until you are ready to begin running. Begin by walking for twenty minutes the first four days, followed by walking for thirty minutes the last four days. If you have no problems with this program, try running for two minutes and walking for

four minutes five times consecutively for a total of thirty minutes. Do this routine three times per week until you feel comfortable. Each week add one minute to the running time and subtract one minute from the walking time until you are running comfortably for the full thirty minutes.

BE SMART AND SAFE

Now that you can run for thirty minutes, do not concern yourself with pace or distance. Gradual training is the key to long-term success, and rest time is just as important as the time you spend training. Be sure to have proper running shoes that suit your individual needs, and be aware of the surface you are running on as well. The best running surface is a track. If you do not have access to a track, asphalt is better than concrete, and dirt or silt alongside the road is even better. From the novice to the expert runner, a local 5k race is a great way to get in shape and improve your sense of health and well-being.

SUPPORT YOUR COMMUNITY

Since running is relatively inexpensive and a great way to stay in shape, the popularity of 5k races has dramatically increased over the past few years. By running a 5k and donating money through your entry fee, you are supporting a larger cause and meeting new people who share similar interests and goals.

PLYOMETRICS: CONTROLLED IMPACT/MAXIMUM POWER

It may sound like the latest Van Damme film, but controlled impact and maximum power are the aims of a training technique called "plyometrics." Also known as jump training, plyometrics involves stretching the muscles prior to contracting them. This type of training, when used safely and effectively, strengthens muscles, increases vertical jump, and decreases impact forces on the joints.

Plyometrics mimics the motions we use in sports such as skiing, tennis, and basketball. If you enjoy dodging moguls, chasing down ground strokes, or charging the net, plyometrics might be an appropriate training option for you. These exercises are designed to increase muscular power and explosiveness. Plyo-

metrics are not for those who are in poor condition or have orthopedic limitations.

OLYMPIC SECRETS

The Eastern Europeans first used plyometrics in the 1970s to develop greater strength and power in their Olympic athletes. They based their programs on scientific evidence that stretching muscles prior to contracting them recruits the "myotactic" or stretch reflex to enhance the power of contraction.

This prestretching of muscles occurs when you perform jumps one after the other. For example, when you land from a jump, the quadricep muscles on the front of your thigh stretch as your knee bends and then quickly contract with the next leap. This prestretch enhances the power of the second jump.

PROCEED WITH CAUTION

Plyometric training has received its share of criticism due to reported cases of injuries following plyometric programs of depth jumping and drop jumping, which involve jumping up to, and down from, boxes or benches that are as high as forty-two inches. The forces sustained from these types of jumps onto hard surfaces can be as much as seven times one's own body weight. However, carefully considering the type of jumps selected for the program, enlisting a coach or trainer for supervision, and gradually increasing to more difficult exercises can make a plyometric program both safe and effective.

Jumps should always begin from the ground level, off and onto padded surfaces such as grass or a gym mat over a wooden gym floor. These types of jumps are both safe and easy to perform. Other training techniques include jumping over cones or foam barriers.

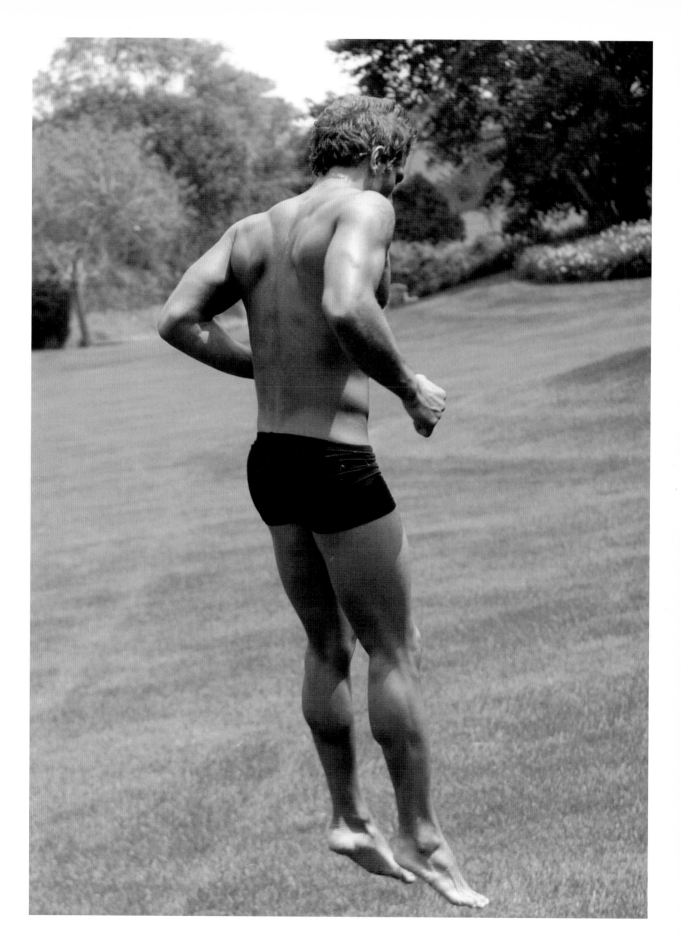

One study found that participants in a well-designed program of stretching, plyometric training, and weight training reduced their landing forces from a jump by 20 percent and increased their hamstring strength by 44 percent. Both of these factors contribute to reducing an individual's potential risk of injury. In addition, some studies have shown plyometrics to have a positive effect on bone density in younger participants.

USE THIS TOOL WISELY

If you are considering plyometrics, proceed with caution. A sports medicine physician or therapist can advise you on whether or not this training technique is suitable for you and may even help you get started, or recommend someone who can. But if improving athletic performance is not a high priority, the additional risk associated with this activity may not be worth the potential benefits.

You will have a more rewarding training experience if you follow the recommendations outlined above. Please use only simple ground-level jumps from soft surfaces, and train under proper supervision. Plyometric training can be a smart addition to a healthy individual's training program as long as it is used wisely.

QUALITY, NOT QUANTITY

A safe and effective plyometric program stresses quality not quantity of jumps. Safe landing techniques, such as landing from toe to heel from a vertical jump and using the entire foot as a rocker to dissipate landing forces over a greater surface area are also important to reduce impact forces. In addition, visualization cues, such as picturing yourself landing "light as a feather"

and "recoiling like a spring" after impact, promote low-impact landings. When landing, avoid excessive side-to-side motion at the knee. Landing forces can be absorbed through the knee musculature (quadriceps, hamstrings, gastrocnemius, or calf muscle) more effectively when the knee is bending primarily in only one plane of motion.

SPIN CYCLE

Cycling is a competitive endurance sport that strips your body of fat, shredding your physique into that lean, sculpted body you work and aim for. Cycling isn't just a "get on your bike and ride" skill. This type of strenuous workout entails more than that. Cycling involves both physical and mental skills, powerful legs, well-developed abdominal muscles, a healthy lower back, as well as focus, commitment, and respect for the road.

Being out on the road can be a religious experience for some men who feel cycling is a "Zen" sport that is singular, meditative, and challenging. Outside of the physical requirements, cycling requires skill and meticulous form just as any other sport does: how to hold your hands, posture, and spinal alignment; the position of the seat; the weight of the legs as they press through each revolution of the pedals. Taking all of these things into consideration and making all of these components work in harmony is what every well-trained cyclist enjoys.

There are a lot of variables to consider when you take up this sport. The kind of cycle to ride (both price and quality), the safety equipment to use (helmets, gloves, eye gear, shorts, etc.), and the types of paths or terrain you are going to ride on. There are several options, both urban and rural. Rural cycling hasn't changed all that much in the past few years. You still have traditional biking along winding roads and distance riding, as well as mountain biking and racing. But the urban scene is where you find some interesting developments.

Cycling has come in from the real world and into the health club by way of Spinning. An indoor group activity now offered in health clubs around the world, spinning was developed by Johnny G., a world-class cyclist based in Los Angeles (I truly admire this visionary and am glad to call him a friend). Spinning is an indoor experience that simulates an outdoor ride performed through a variety of terrain and at varying speeds. Visualization and imagination add a degree of intensity that only you can create in your head.

Anyone who trains at this level would ultimately hope to get out on the road. Any professional instructor who teaches this type of cycling class in any club would love to see people get out on the road and enjoy the sport of cycling in its purest form.

Product developers and marketing managers will always try to capture your dollar by way of introducing you to the newest, greatest, most technologically advanced training method. If all of that intimidates you, then just get on a Lifecycle or exercise bike that can increase resistance to the legs. Change the resistance every three or four minutes from light to heavy to intermediate. This is how indoor cycling resembles the outdoor ride. When the resistance is high, it is like riding up a steep hill. When the resistance is low, it is like riding on a flat surface and you are gliding along with speed and rhythm. Use what is available to you or go out and get the tools or take a class. Try it!

Tip: If you do choose to start riding and want the upper hand on how hard your legs will have to work, train them with Lunges. Lunges will challenge your legs enough to get stronger, more powerful legs and will add balance, which is something that you will have to do on a bike when you stand up out of the saddle to climb those high hills.

TIME

How often have you heard (or used!) the excuse, "I don't have time to exercise?" Most people believe that the only way to improve fitness is to put aside a chunk of time to devote just to exercise. These people neglect to take advantage of bits of time available throughout the day to exercise. These snippets of time will add up to a significant amount of time by the end of the day and will add to your overall fitness while helping to lower your stress level.

Here are some ideas, many of which you have probably heard before:

- Park at the far end of the parking lot and walk briskly to your destination.

- While brushing your teeth, alternate balancing on one foot.

- Wear fitness shoes to work; when you take a break, take a walk.

- While driving, concentrate on pulling your abdominals in tight.

- For errands close by, walk or ride your bicycle.

- While on hold on the telephone, stand and do some lunges or squats.

- When alone in an elevator, do some wall push-ups.

- While sitting anywhere, practice proper posture to avoid back pain.

- Take the stairs instead of the elevator. For one floor, slowly take two stairs at a time, pushing up through the heel.

- While watching TV, do some floor exercises (leg lifts, abdominal crunches, etc.) or relaxing stretches.

- Jump rope for five minutes.

- While cooking, do some calf raises and glute squeezes.

- Carry your own groceries to the car.

- While cleaning the house, alternate using each hand to work arms evenly.

- While your kids are playing at the park, go along and play with them!

Use these ideas and add some of your own. Start thinking of fitness as important enough to occupy a set time frame in your week. Make a commitment to yourself to start adding up your exercise minutes throughout the day, every day.

MINIMALIST WORKOUT

These six exercises can work all of the body's major muscle groups at home or at the gym. All you need are two or three sets or dumbbells (try ten- to twenty-pound weights) and a bench or ball.

A few key tips:

- Warm up for five minutes with light cardiovascular exercise, such as brisk walking in place, before lifting.

- Perform sets of eight to twelve repetitions. Choose weights heavy enough so that the last rep is a real struggle (but not so much of one that you're forced to contort your body). You may need to use a different amount of weight for each exercise. With some of the moves, your body weight may be enough, so you might not need to add a dumbbell.

- Perform each exercise with controlled movements, taking a full two seconds to get to the extreme position and a full two seconds to return to the starting position. Rely on muscle power not momentum.

- Rest no more than thirty seconds between exercises.

THE MOVES

PUSH-UP (WORKS THE CHEST, TRICEPS, AND FRONT OF THE SHOULDER). Kneel with your ankles crossed or legs extended straight out behind you, arms straight, palms on the floor a bit to the side and in front of your shoulders, and your face to the floor. Bend your elbows and lower your body until your upper arms are parallel to the floor. Keep your abs tight and pelvis tucked at all times so your back doesn't sag. Push back up. For the advanced version of the push-up, put a stability ball under your feet or under your hands.

ONE-ARM ROW (STRENGTHENS THE BACK, BICEPS, AND BACK OF THE SHOULDER). Place a ball or a bench in front of you. Holding a dumbbell in your right hand, stand with your right foot on the floor and your left knee touching the ball. Lean forward and place your left hand on the ball in front of you. Keep your back straight and abs tight with your right knee slightly bent. Your right arm should hang straight down. Bend your elbow, lifting the dumbbell until your elbow is higher than your back and your hand

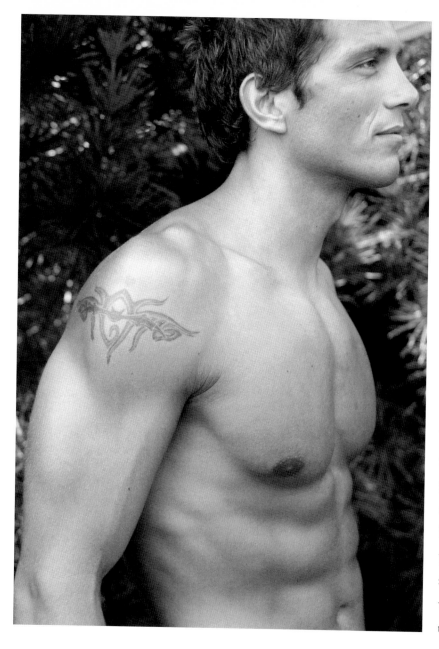

each hand, stand with your feet hip-width apart, knees slightly bent, and abs tucked in. Raise your upper arms to shoulder height so that the dumbbells are at ear level. Push the dumbbells up and in until the ends of the weights are nearly touching directly over your head. Then lower the dumbbells back to ear level.

WALL SQUAT (WORKS THE BUT-TOCKS, QUADRICEPS, AND HAM-STRINGS). Hold a dumbbell in each hand or place your hands on your hips or on the tops of your thighs. Stand up tall against the ball, ball against the wall positioned in the middle of your back with your abs tight, feet hip-width apart, and your weight slightly back on your heels. Sit down, as if you're sitting into a chair. Don't squat any lower than the point at which your thighs are parallel to the floor, and don't let your knees shoot out in front of your toes.

brushes against your waist. Lower the weight slowly back down. After completing the reps with your right arm, switch sides. To advance—as you lift each arm from the elbow, rotate your upper body to the same side until you can see the ceiling. As you lower the weight, rotate back to your starting position.

Stand back up. To advance—start up the weight or slow down the sit to a crawl.

DUMBBELL SHOULDER PRESS (WORKS THE FRONT AND MIDDLE SHOULDERS). Holding a dumbbell in

LUNGE (WORKS THE BUTTOCKS, QUADRICEPS, HAMSTRINGS, AND CALVES). Hold a dumbbell in each hand or place your hands on your hips. Stand tall with your abs tight, feet hip-width apart, and weight back on your heels. Lift your right toe slightly and, leading with your heel, step your right foot forward

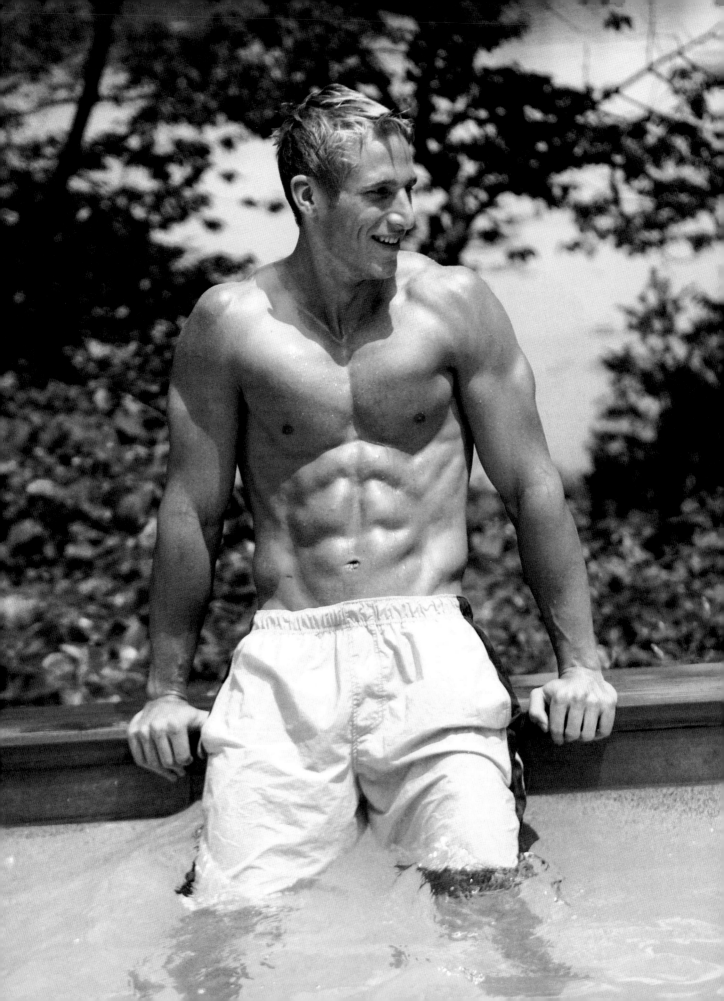

about a stride's length. As your foot touches the floor, bend both knees until your right thigh is parallel to the floor and your left thigh is perpendicular to it. Your left heel will lift off the floor. Push back to the standing position. To advance—step forward instead of pushing back and continue walking forward for twenty steps.

BALL CRUNCH (WORKS THE ABDOMINALS). Lie on the ball with your knees bent and feet flat on the floor hip-width apart. Place your hands behind your head so your thumbs are behind your ears, without lacing your fingers together. Hold your elbows out to the sides but rounded slightly in. Tilt your chin slightly toward your chest and tighten your abs. Curl up and forward so that your head, neck, and shoulder blades lift off the floor. Hold for a moment and then lower slowly back down.

Designing an exercise program isn't rocket science. Mixing it up a bit might be the key for you. The *minimum* requirements should include:

- **Resistance training.** Two days a week, eight to twelve exercises covering major muscles of the upper and lower body.

- **Flexibility.** Stretch major muscle groups four times a week, hold each stretch thirty seconds.

- **Cardiovascular exercise.** Three days of aerobic fitness training for a minimum of twenty minutes at a target heart rate of 60 to 80 percent (85 to 90 percent for the highly fit.)

MORE MINIMALIST WORKOUTS

Here are four sample fitness plans. Remember to check with your doctor before beginning this or any other exercise program.

Begin each plan with a five- to ten-minute warm-up and end with a three- to five-minute cooldown, followed by stretches for calves, Achilles tendons, hamstrings, quadriceps, chest, shoulders, neck, and the middle, lower, and upper back.

Beginners, keep your total workout times—including warm-up, cooldown, and stretches—to about thirty-five minutes. Progressively increase time or intensity as you become stronger.

BASIC TRAINING. Total time: forty-five to sixty minutes, three days a week. Twenty minutes of any aerobic activity, such as walking, jogging, swimming, aerobic dance, or cycling. Three sets (eight to twelve repetitions) of resistance-training exercises. Choose one exercise for each muscle group.

CIRCUIT TRAINING. Try this variation on basic training: Spend two minutes performing any aerobic activity, such as walking. Immediately follow the aerobic exercise with a resistance exercise—for example, one minute of Wall Squats. Go back to another aerobic activity for two minutes and continue the circuit.

INTERVAL TRAINING. Add power bursts to your aerobic activity. Every three minutes or so during your aerobic workout, add a one-minute "power interval" to increase intensity. For example, walk at 3.5 mph for three minutes, then try walking at 4 mph for one minute before returning to your 3.5 mph pace. Repeat.

CROSS TRAINING. Bored? Try something different. Take a boxing or yoga class. If you always ride the stationary bike, try the treadmill. You can also break up your work-out time with a fitness buffet. That is, ride the bike for ten minutes, jump rope for five minutes, walk on the treadmill for ten minutes, then try five minutes of stair climbing. Still not inspired? Buy a new fitness video or work out with a friend.

Start with the minimum requirements and an attainable goal for yourself. Find success this way and then move on to a new goal. Most important, make the commitment to yourself to do it.

HOME CIRCUIT

Working out at home and performing the same exercise routine every day can lose its appeal. Fortunately, initiating modest changes in the way you exercise can enhance motivation. Why not liven up your workouts with a homemade circuit? Circuit training involves visiting a series of stations, each intended to target different muscles and exercises. Circuits are a cinch to organize and require only a few pieces of key equipment. And a circuit format can facilitate crosstraining by allowing you to easily incorporate a variety of new moves.

You can organize a circuit with existing home gym equipment by creating a resistance circuit using inexpensive tubing, handheld weights, and a stability ball. If you have one or more cardio machines, consider a combination muscular endurance and cardio circuit. Alternate between several stations of muscular endurance and longer cardio sessions. Or complete your cardio and then carry out a resistance-training circuit.

You can also achieve a total body workout using only a stability ball and your own body weight. Exercises like push-ups, squats, abdominal curls, and calf raises are simple and effective with a ball.

Be imaginative, but exercise caution. Obviously, avoid breakable bottles, sharp objects, or unstable furniture. Creating a circuit at home requires special attention to safety measures. Avoid propulsive movements like ski jumps or skipping on a slippery carpet, floor, or concrete surface. Make sure you have a clear, open space to assemble stations. Be prepared to temporarily move furniture aside. If you have limited space, consider a fixed circuit that doesn't require movement from station to station. If you opt for a stationary setup, remember to clear unnecessary equipment out of the way before each new drill.

Choosing an appropriate time to spend at each station will depend on your fitness goals and the circuit's focus. Plan for most drills to last anywhere from thirty seconds to several minutes, or even longer for cardio segments. You may find that a thirty-second period is too short for some exercises, but several minutes is too long for others. Play with the timing until you find a time span that is appropriate for your needs and level. Allow ten to fifteen seconds for travel between stations.

FIVE TOP FITNESS TIPS

Every year, millions of Americans vow to join the ranks of fitness buffs, yet more than 60 percent of adults are not regularly active and 25 percent are not active at all. It's not that we're ignorant—we know that exercise is important. Its benefits are touted everywhere. Regular exercise reduces the risk of heart disease, diabetes, high blood pressure, and colon cancer. It also enhances mental health. But working out sounds like, well, just too much work.

How can you overcome this hurdle? Discuss your plan with your doctor, and then take it one tiny step at a time. Think of the fable of the tortoise and the hare: A moderate pace and consistent behavior win the race. A quick fix may get you ahead for a few weeks, but it doesn't provide the overall effects of a safe, regular exercise routine.

ASSESS YOUR FITNESS LEVEL AND SET GOALS. Are you a couch potato or a weekend athlete? Do you want to get fit in order to live longer or to tone your body? Just thirty minutes of walking each day will improve your health, but you'll need more if you want to build muscle.

FIND THE RIGHT EXERCISE FOR YOU. One of the best ways to stick with exercise is to find one you enjoy. What are your preferences? What styles of exercise suit you? And once you've figured that out, how do you find fitness programs in your community? What about choosing a health club or personal trainer?

CARDIOVASCULAR EXERCISE: HOW MUCH? When it comes to cardiovascular or aerobic exercise, you've got some choices to make: long duration and mild intensity—such as walking or swimming—or short duration and high intensity—such as running or climbing stairs quickly. Both will strengthen your heart and burn fat. And although intensity aerobics will burn more fat in less time, in order to get your body and heart conditioned, you need to mix it up a bit.

RESISTANCE TRAINING AND FLEXIBILITY WORK: WHY? Strength training, such as lifting hand or leg weights, preserves bone density, increases muscle mass, and improves strength and balance. Flexibility exercises, such as stretching, help warm you up and pre-vent injuries. It's important to build both into your workout. You don't need to buy fancy equipment. You can start by lifting a one-pound can of food.

DESIGN A PROGRAM AND STAY MOTIVATED. You can design a program for a total workout, and you can stick to it. Set aside just half an hour each day. You'll feel better—for life!

SHAKING UP YOUR WEIGHT TRAINING

When it comes to working out, many of us are creatures of habit. We do what we know. We stick with what's familiar and comfortable. The catch is that if you always do the same thing the same way, your body will adapt, and your results will grind to a halt. This is especially true of strength training, where you need to keep your body guessing if you want to keep seeing results. Here are some techniques for breaking through strength-training plateaus and keeping the results coming:

EXERCISE VARIETY

It's important to regularly vary the exercises you do and the order in which you do them. Different moves recruit muscle fibers in different ways. By varying your routine, you keep your muscles changing and adapting, and therefore you keep seeing results. Keep in mind that machine exercises tend to isolate the working muscle, while free-weight exercises incorporate additional muscle groups for balance and stability. They both have advantages. Try to find several good exercises for each body part and alternate them regularly.

PREEXHAUST

In addition to trying new exercises, experiment with their order. If you've always worked large muscle groups and compound movements first, experiment with preexhaust by doing isolation movements first. For example, by first working (preexhausting) your quadriceps on a leg-extension machine, you can force your hamstrings and glutes to do more of the work on squats or leg presses. Be sure to proceed cautiously, and always use a spotter for heavy or difficult movements.

SLOW LIFTING

Step into any weight room and you're almost guaranteed to see someone struggling with way too much weight, jerky movements, and very poor form. Quite a few people are guilty of compromising good form in an attempt to lift heavier weights. If you've reached what seems like the upper limit of your capabilities, try taking a few plates off of your weight load and performing the same movement very, very slowly—try ten counts on the lifting movement and four counts on the lowering movement. By moving slowly and precisely through the full range of motion, you totally eliminate momentum, increase tension on the working muscle, and recruit all kinds of additional muscle fibers. You'll feel it! Be sure to cut back on the number of repetitions when training this way. Your muscle is going to fatigue much more quickly.

BREAKDOWN TRAINING

In a nutshell, this means that once you've worked a muscle to failure, you reduce the load and crank out a few more repetitions with a lighter weight. Suppose that you normally do leg curls with seventy pounds of resistance, and that you reach muscle failure after ten repetitions. Rather than stopping at the end of the set, you would reduce the weight to sixty pounds and immediately perform two or three additional reps. This is another excellent way to up the intensity of the exercise and recruit additional muscle fibers.

ASSISTED TRAINING

This concept is very similar to breakdown training, but it requires the help of a partner. Once you reach the point of failure on a particular exercise, your partner steps in and assists you with the movement. So if after ten barbell biceps curls, you can't complete another repetition with good form, your partner steps in and helps you lift the bar to the top of the movement. This allows you to perform two or three postfatigue repetitions, again upping the intensity and promoting further strength gains.

NEGATIVE TRAINING

This can be approached from two slightly different angles, both of which emphasize the eccentric or lowering phase of the exercise. One option is to carefully lower more weight than you can lift (with the assistance of a qualified trainer or spotter). For example, if you're not strong enough to do chin-ups, you can have a trainer assist you to the top of the movement and then you slowly lower your own body weight. The other option is to simply emphasize the lowering portion of the exercise by slowing it down several counts. Either way, you're working the muscle in a different way, incorporating additional muscle fibers and promoting strength gains.

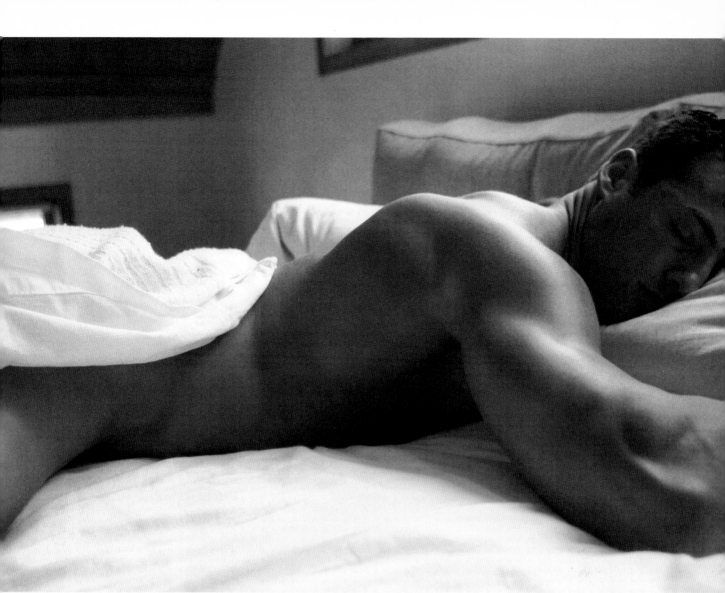

PERIODIZATION

The idea is to avoid always using the same workload. One way to accomplish this is to set up a program of planned periodization. For example, you might do three weeks of multiple-set, high-repetition endurance training, followed by three weeks of increased weight and fewer repetitions, followed by three weeks of very heavy single-set exercises, followed by a week off. Then you would repeat the pattern. There are numerous ways to approach periodization, but the basic idea is to keep changing the intensity at regular intervals so that your workouts don't stagnate.

REST

A final reminder here. Many of these techniques can greatly increase the intensity of your workouts. As the intensity increases, so does your need for rest and recovery time. Remember that your muscles don't actually grow while you're training. They grow during the rest period between workouts. If you don't allow enough recovery time between workouts, your size and strength gains will be greatly diminished. Be sure to adjust your training schedule accordingly.

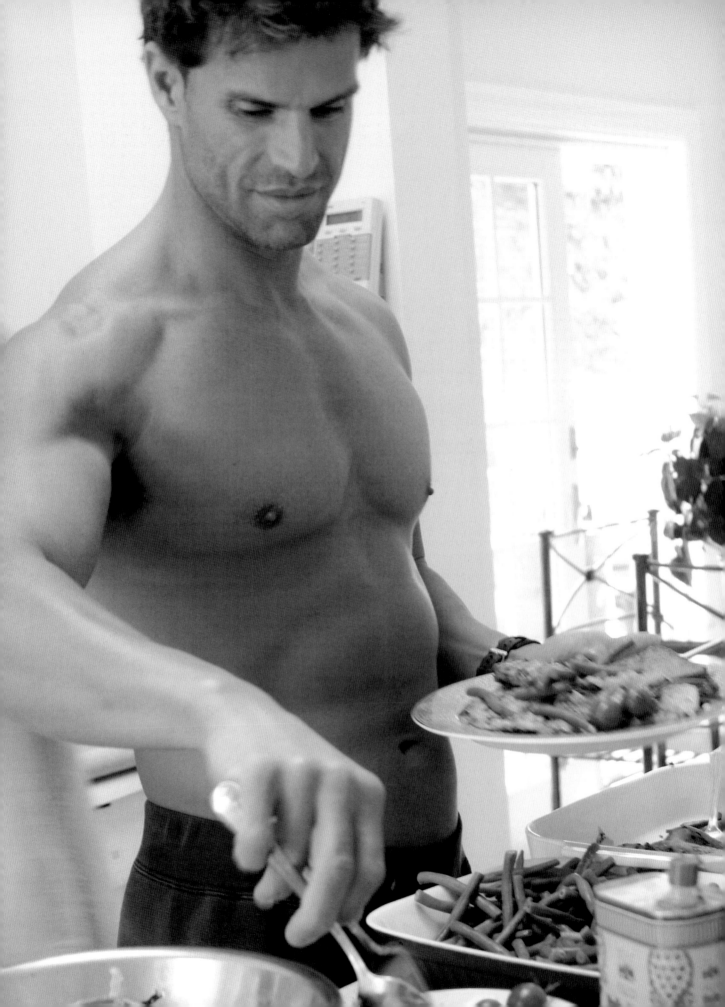

CHAPTER NINE

NUTRITION STRATEGIES

SUCCESSFUL WEIGHT CONTROL

It's not just cutting calories. Eating less, or cutting back on fat in your diet, won't keep the weight off. What you really need to do is strike a good balance between the number of calories you consume and the number you burn. And the only way to do that is to exercise.

Don't groan! By exercising, you can lose weight while you eat more calories than if you simply went on a diet. Regular physical activity is much more effective at keeping weight off in the long run than any diet.

With aerobic exercise, you can lose weight as long as you reduce the calories you consume. One main reason for this is because aerobic exercise elevates your metabolism only while you're exercising, You've probably heard about exercise programs that actually turn your body into a "fat-burning machine." An aerobic program you stick with can help you lose weight more easily because it can stimulate your body and make it burn calories.

If weight control is your goal, some types of aerobic activity will work better than others. Low-impact aerobics, like walking, step aerobics, and low-impact aerobic dance are your best bets. Some good no-impact aerobic activities you can benefit from include swimming, bicycling, and rowing.

If you're just getting started, begin with as little as fifteen minutes of low-impact aerobics three times a week. Gradually increase to thirty minutes of moderate aerobic activity four times a week.

STRENGTH TRAINING = WEIGHT MANAGEMENT

Your muscles burn calories during physical activity. What you may not know is your muscles also burn calories when your body is at rest. Increase your muscle mass, and you'll be increasing your body's capacity to burn calories both during activity and at rest.

Add to that research that shows diets that restrict calories can substantially cause the loss of lean muscle mass, along with the loss of fat. By incorporating strength training into your activity program, as well as following a moderate diet, you'll be able to maintain lean muscle mass while you lose fat.

Start any strength-training program with one set of exercises and a weight that allows you to complete eight to twelve repetitions. Your program should exercise your legs, arms, chest, and upper back. If you want to strengthen your stomach and lower back, increase the number of repetitions with weights that offer less resistance.

Success means good eating and good exercise. Follow a moderate, low-fat diet and an exercise program that combines aerobic activity and strength training. That's the key to losing weight—and keeping it off.

Begin slowly with exercises you find comfortable with and build as your body becomes accustomed to the activity level. Don't start out too hard or too fast. Chances are you may injure yourself or quit before you've done yourself much good.

And remember, you can't lose weight overnight. Set a realistic weight-loss goal for yourself—like one to two pounds a week—eat healthy, get going on a program of regular physical activity, and you'll be delighted by what you accomplish.

Maintaining a lower, healthier body weight is something you can accomplish. So start now and keep on going!

PUTTING ON THE POUNDS

No, you didn't misread the heading. Believe it or not, there are some people who are looking to put pounds on. They want, maybe even need, to gain weight. Since most people spend much of their lives figuring out ways to shed their extra pounds, the concept of underweight may be difficult to comprehend. However, if you're a part of the minority population that has tried everything they can to gain weight, you know that it can be just as difficult for underweight people to add pounds as it is for overweight people to take them off.

WHO NEEDS TO GAIN WEIGHT?

The term *underweight* is generally used to describe two kinds of people: those whose weight is considered below normal, but who are still healthy, and those whose low weights are cause for significant health concerns. The latter group is at high risk for respiratory diseases, tuberculosis, digestive disorders, and some cancers, and women are more likely to become infertile or give birth to unhealthy babies. A consultation with their physicians is recommended for these people before they embark on a program to gain weight.

Individuals in the former category may range from young football players who wish to create a stronger presence on the field to older adults living ordinary lives. These people usually have a genetic predisposition to thinness, and it is important that they keep this in mind when implementing strategies for gaining weight; they won't be able to change their physiology, but they may be able to enhance it.

A useful rule of thumb is that in order to gain one pound of body weight per week, you should consume an additional five hundred calories per day above the amount you typically consume. This number varies from person to person (depending on such factors as weight and metabolism), but you get the idea: Eating more than normal is a must if you want to gain weight. Boost your calories by consistently consuming three larger-than-normal meals a day plus two or more snacks during the midmorning and midafternoon. Try to eat foods that are high in calories, but remember to stay away from saturated fats, such as cheese, beef, butter, and bacon. It's best to stick to a high-carbohydrate, low-fat diet that you modify to include larger quantities. This also applies to your intake of protein. Many athletes seeking to gain muscle use protein powders and amino acid supplements. This isn't necessary if you eat the recommended amount of dietary protein (15 to 20 percent of daily calories), which is less expensive and more effective than buying supplements. To be sure that you are sensibly increasing your caloric intake, make an appointment with a registered dietitian who can help you plan your meals.

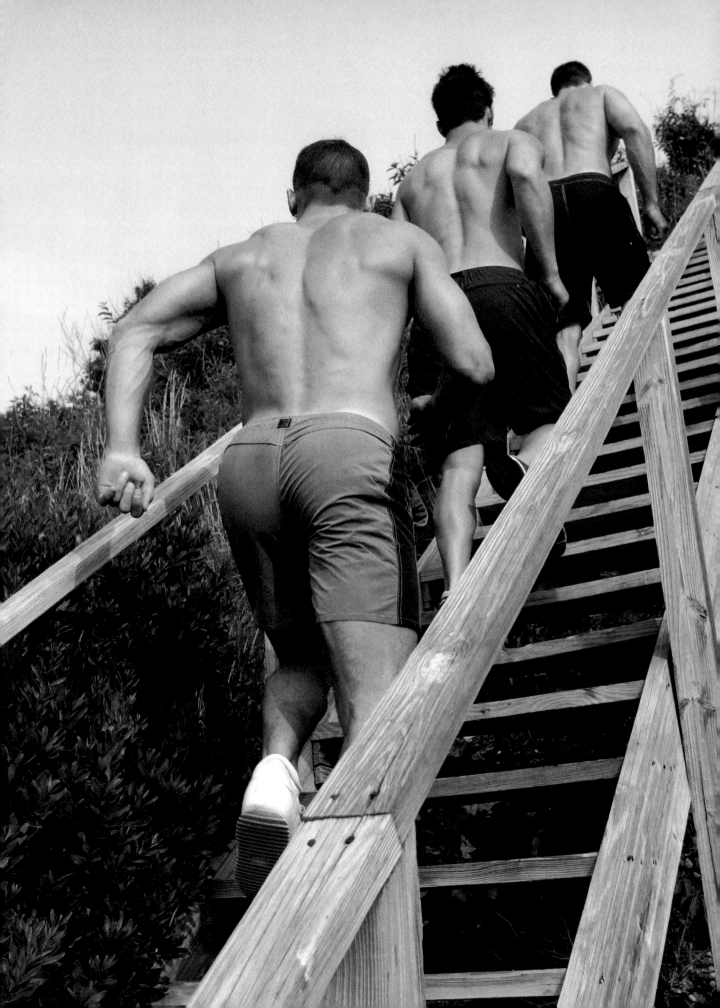

THE KEY

In order to ensure that the extra calories you are eating don't simply turn into gained pounds of fat, it is crucial that you make strength training your primary form of exercise. If you rely only on eating calorie-dense foods to gain weight, you will only gain fat—not likely the change you are looking for. Strength training will convert the extra calories you consume into muscle growth that will enhance your appearance as well as your performance in daily activities and athletics. Working with an American Council on Exercise (ACE) certified personal trainer is a good way to learn which strength-training exercises will be best for you and to make sure that you are performing them correctly. (Call 800-529-8227 to locate the ACE-certified personal trainer nearest you.)

BE PATIENT

Putting on weight can be a hard and often slow task, but if you consistently eat large meals and participate in strength training, the payoff should be worth both the wait and the work.

KEEP IT SIMPLE

The secret to good nutrition and eating well is remarkably simple: be careful of your calorie intake and eat lots of fruits and vegetables. There is no shortcut to a healthy lifestyle; we all know what it takes to eat right, and we all know that just a little discipline will help get us there.

The growing interest in nutrition has seemingly elevated nutritional experts to the level of demigods in our culture. People are willing to believe any piece of information that could potentially hold the key to better living, and unfortunately this willingness has led to a number of misconceptions about nutrition. Here are some frequently asked questions followed by answers to help you debunk some health mysteries.

Q. *Should I be taking a vitamin and mineral supplement if I eat well?*

A. By eating a balanced diet that incorporates all four food groups with consistent servings of fruits and vegetables, you will consume all the vitamins and minerals your body requires. A vitamin supplement will provide no additional benefit to your health unless you're suffering from some kind of deficiency. As well, people who do not follow a good diet (those who eat an abundance of dairy, bread, and meat) should take a supplement to help offset some deficiencies. Pills cannot replace all the nutrients that come from food. For your body to function properly, you need to make a concerted effort to eat more vitamin-rich foods like vegetables and fruit.

Q. *What are some healthy snacks besides fruits and vegetables?*

A. When preparing a snack, try to choose from one of the four food groups: grains; vegetables and fruit; dairy; or meat and high-protein alternatives. Some great options include a cut-up banana wrapped in a pita with peanut butter on it or an apple and cheese. Mixing some granola with yogurt also makes for a healthy snack. Anything that incorporates a majority of the food groups is a healthy alternative to anything you'll find in the snack aisle of the supermarket.

Q. *Will eating late at night lead to weight gain?*

A. The common assumption is that eating late at night will not give your body the chance to burn off the calories, and you will gain weight. The truth is that your body processes calories the same way at night as during the day. The problem with late-night eating is that people tend to indulge in junk food rather than something healthy, and that is what leads to weight gain.

Q. *Can carbohydrates make me fat?*

A. Yes and no. With a number of very trendy diets preaching the merits of cutting carbohydrates from your diet, the world now seems to think that they are the source of all fat. The misconception arises because generally carbohydrates turn to glucose in your body. Any glucose not used by the cells gets converted and stored as glycogen in the muscles and liver, and the excess is converted into fat. So while carbohydrates are not terrible, they should be consumed in moderation.

Q. *Should I have a protein shake after training?*

A. Much as with vitamin supplements, you need to examine your protein intake and whether or not it is adequate. The average male requires around fifty-nine to sixty-five grams of protein per day to remain healthy. If, however, you are interested in increasing your muscle mass or gaining weight, then adding more protein to your diet via a shake is one way to do so.

Q. *Is soda bad for me?*

A. Nutritionists will tell you over and over again that weight gain is the result of high caloric intake and low physical activity. Most sodas are filled with sugar, which ultimately means high calorie content, and in order to burn those calories you have to exercise. If you don't, the calories will be stored as fat, and you will start to gain weight.

Q. *Should I stop drinking coffee?*

A. Coffee has become a vice that everyone wants to be rid of in theory but with no real motivation to quit. The only real negative side effect of coffee comes from the overconsumption of caffeine. Ingesting large amounts of the stimulant can cause an increase in alertness, heart rate, and blood pressure, not to mention leading to sleep deprivation. Other than that, no study has shown any problems related directly to the drinking of coffee. But watch your calorie intake when it comes to gourmet coffees, iced coffees, and café au laits, as they have high levels of sugar and cream.

Q. *Are foods labeled "low fat" better for me?*

A. The label itself serves as more of a marketing tool than a health service. You should not assume that "low fat" equates to "healthy"—especially considering that low-fat products tend to be high in carbohydrates and processed sugar. If you are trying to lose weight, however, the low-fat or fat-free version of a product will generally contain fewer calories than the regular version. But don't let that give you an incentive to consume double the portion.

Q. *Is it healthy to eat red meat?*

A. Red meat is one of those things that doctors recommend we cut from our diet as we get older, and in recent years, it has been stigmatized as a trouble food. In reality, it is loaded with nutrients, including iron and protein, which are essential for muscle growth. Eating lean meat in moderation is part of a healthy diet.

Q. *Is it better to eat small meals every two to three hours rather than three big meals per day?*

A. The answer to this question really depends on your goals. If weight loss is your objective, then five small meals throughout the day may be the best way to do it. This will help jump-start your metabolism and increase your body's ability to burn fat.

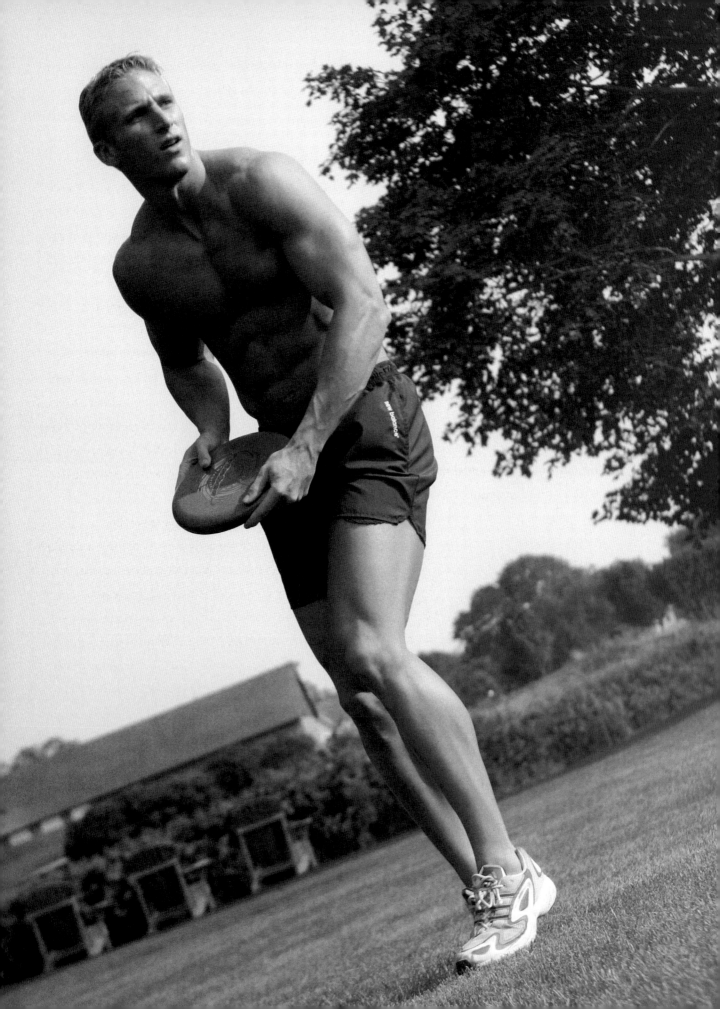

Q. *Is drinking tea good for me?*

A. This question is still in the early stages of receiving a proper answer from scientists. Currently, studies are generally reporting that drinking green tea is good for the body. Its main nutritional benefit comes from "antioxidants," which help prevent cholesterol in the blood from becoming oxidized, which is believed to lead to heart disease.

WEIGHT-LOSS PLATEAUS AND PITFALLS

It's kind of like running into a wall—that feeling you get when, after a few months on a weight-loss program, you suddenly stop seeing results. This is called hitting a plateau, and it is not uncommon. In fact, unless you continually update your program to reflect the changes your body has already experienced, you can almost be guaranteed to plateau at some point along your journey toward reaching your goal weight.

WEIGHT-LOSS WOES

The first thing you should do when you hit a plateau is try to determine the cause. Could you be eating more calories than you think? Research shows that most people underreport the number of calories they eat. It's not that they're lying, they just don't know how to make an accurate assessment of how much they're eating. And even if you're eating fewer calories than before you lost the weight, you could be eating just enough to maintain your current weight at your current activity level. It is important to keep in mind that as you lose weight, your metabolism slows down because there is less of you to fuel, both at rest and during activity. So while a diet of eighteen hundred calories per day helped you lose a certain amount of weight, if you've hit a plateau, it could be that eigh-teen hundred calories is the exact amount you need to stay at your current weight.

EXERCISE YOUR OPTIONS

This leaves you with two options: Lower your caloric intake further or increase the amount of time you spend being physically active. The first option is less desirable because you may not be able to get sufficient nutrients from a diet that is very low in calories, and it is difficult to stick to it for very long. It is much better to moderately reduce calories to a level that you can sustain when you reach your goal weight. The same is true for exercise. Trying to exercise for several hours per day to burn more calories is a good way to set yourself up for failure. Not only does this type of reg-imen require an enormous time commitment, but it's hard on the body, making you more susceptible to in-jury and overuse syndromes.

To help balance intake with expenditure, a good rule of thumb is to multiply your goal weight by ten calories per pound and add more calories according to how active you are. Again, be realistic. Don't attempt too much in an effort to burn more calories. Instead, aim for thirty minutes of moderate activity most of the days of the week, and as you become more fit, gradually increase the intensity and duration of your exercise sessions. Choose activities that you find enjoy-able, whether that be in-line skating, step classes, or even mall walking.

Another means for getting you off a plateau is strength training, which has been shown to be very effec-tive in helping people manage their weight because the added muscle helps to offset the metabolism-lowering ef-fect of dieting and losing weight. Muscle is much more metabolically active than fat; therefore, the more muscle you can add, the higher your metabolism will be.

GET OFF THE PLATEAU

If you've stopped losing weight, the key to getting off the plateau is to vary your program. The human body is an amazing piece of machinery, capable of adapting to just about any circumstance or stimulus. By shaking things up a bit and varying your program by introducing some new elements, you'll likely find yourself off the plateau and back on the road to progress in no time.

CALORIE BURNERS: ACTIVITIES THAT TURN UP THE HEAT

When it comes to burning calories, most of us want to get as much mileage out of our exercise as possible. For many, the more calories we burn, the better we feel about our workout. While energy expenditure should not be the only measure of a good workout (remember, it's good for you and makes you feel pretty good, too), it is helpful to know what a given activity might be costing you in terms of calories.

A word of caution, though, about counting calories. Simply burning more calories will take you only so far down the road to better health. A well-balanced, low-fat diet, plenty of rest, and a healthy attitude are also essential. And, of course, all things in moderation—even exercise.

READING THIS CHART

The numbers on the chart on page 157 correspond to how many calories individuals of various weights burn per minute during different activities. Simply multiply this number by how many minutes you perform a given activity. For example, a 160-pound man jogging will burn about 12.4 calories per minute or 372 calories during a thirty-minute jog.

There are a few things you should keep in mind as you review this chart. With exercise, it really is true that you get out of it what you put into it. Simply showing up for class and going through the motions isn't going to do you much good. To get the most out of your exercise session, give it your all, even if your all is less than what others might be doing.

And don't forget to look for little ways to increase the number of calories you burn each day. You might be surprised to learn that it is possible to burn more calories simply by becoming more active in your daily life. Doing things like taking the stairs, walking to the mailbox instead of driving, and doing chores around the house are great ways to burn additional calories.

ACTIVITY CALORIES/MIN.	120 LB.	140 LB.	160 LB.	180 LB.
Basketball	7.5	8.8	10.0	11.3
Bowling	1.2	1.4	1.6	1.9
Cycling (10 mph)	5.5	6.4	7.3	8.2
Dancing (aerobic)	7.4	8.6	9.8	11.1
Dancing (social)	2.9	3.3	3.7	4.2
Gardening	5.0	5.9	6.7	7.5
Golf (pull/carry clubs)	4.6	5.4	6.2	7.0
Golf (power cart)	2.1	2.5	2.8	3.2
Hiking	4.5	5.2	6.0	6.7
Jogging	9.3	10.8	12.4	13.9
Running	11.4	13.2	15.1	17.0
Sitting, quietly	1.2	1.3	1.5	1.7
Skating (ice and roller)	5.9	6.9	7.9	8.8
Skiing (cross-country)	7.5	8.8	10.0	11.3
Skiing (water/downhill)	5.7	6.6	7.6	8.5
Swimming (crawl)	7.8	9.0	10.3	11.6
Tennis	6.0	6.9	7.9	8.9
Walking	6.5	7.6	8.7	9.7
Weight training	6.6	7.6	8.7	9.8

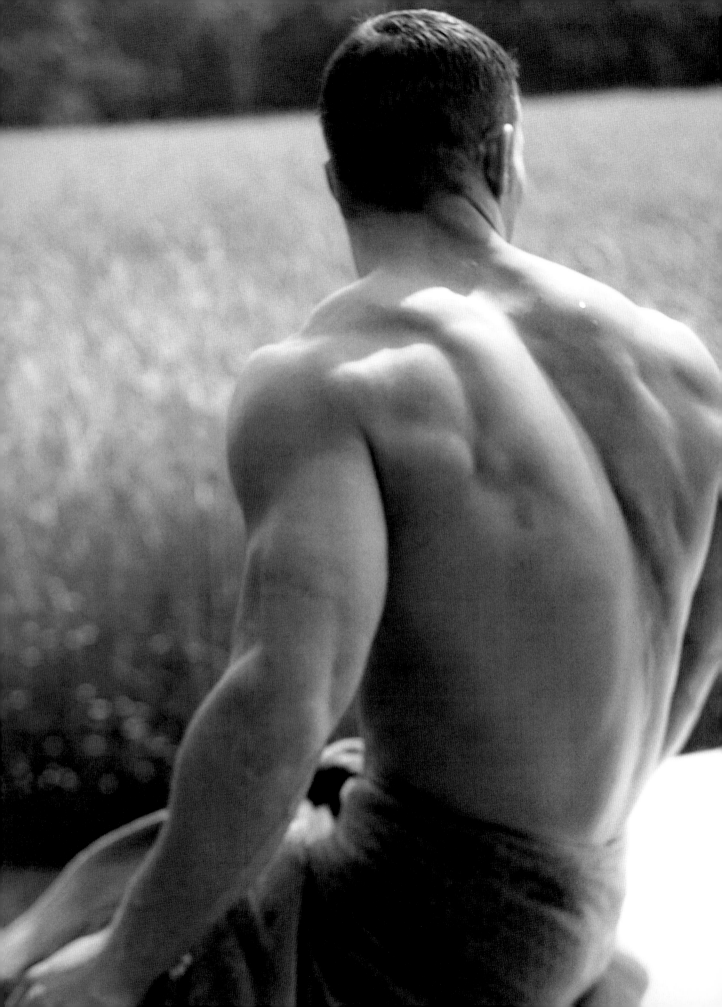

Change your focus from weight loss to weight management. You may also need to change your unhealthy relationship with food. Weight management includes eating and activity habits that reduce your risk for certain diseases. Use the following ABCs for good health as simple guidelines for your success.

AIM FOR FITNESS

Normally, cardiovascular endurance and muscle strength decline after the age of thirty by about 1 percent and 6 percent, respectively. You can slow the speed of decline by being physically active, which includes an exercise program and an active daily life. In addition, regular exercise can improve your blood cholesterol and triglyceride levels, reduce blood sugar, and improve other risk factors for disease.

Aim to be physically active every day. You can still be fit even if you are overweight or obese. In a study of more than 25,000 volunteers, researchers at the Cooper Clinic found that a person's fitness level was a stronger predictor of death risk than body weight. Overweight or obese men in this study who were physically fit had a lower death risk than men who were a healthy weight but were not physically fit.

BUILD A HEALTHY BASE

Develop a better eating strategy. Use the Food Guide Pyramid to design a healthy diet. Eating regular meals is an important part of a healthy diet. Eat at least three to five small meals a day to spread your intake of food throughout the day. Don't skip meals because you will be more likely to overeat during the next meal. Use the following steps to start eating regularly:

- Get out your cookbooks and plan several days' meals at a time. Planned meals tend to be more balanced than food grabbed on the run. Make a list of the menus and post it on your refrigerator.

- Make a grocery list of what you need to buy to prepare the meals. Add any necessary staples (such as salt, bread, or milk) to your list. Buy only the items on your list. You can save money by not making impulsive purchases.

- The rewards of menu planning are worth it, and you will become more skilled at planning meals with practice. Save your menus and grocery lists and use them again.

CHOOSE SENSIBLY

If you have been struggling with your weight, you may have developed some poor eating habits. You may have negative ideas about food. Many people classify foods as "good" and "bad" based on their

FOOD GUIDE PYRAMID

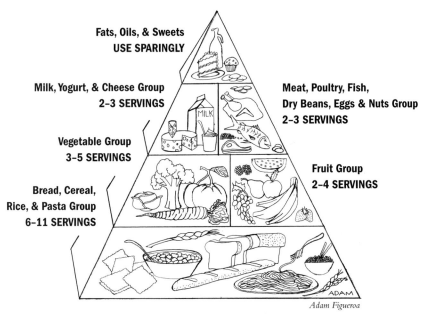

Fats, Oils, & Sweets
USE SPARINGLY

Milk, Yogurt, & Cheese Group
2–3 SERVINGS

Meat, Poultry, Fish,
Dry Beans, Eggs & Nuts Group
2–3 SERVINGS

Vegetable Group
3–5 SERVINGS

Fruit Group
2–4 SERVINGS

Bread, Cereal,
Rice, & Pasta Group
6–11 SERVINGS

Adam Figueroa

calorie content and, sometimes, their nutrient content. All kinds of foods can fit into a healthy diet.

Here are some tips for choosing your food sensibly:

- Watch your portions. Learn what equals a serving for each of the food groups and make sure you are not eating larger portions than the recommended number of servings. Try eating portions the size of your palm.

- Eat low-fat foods. A low-fat diet (less than 30 percent of calories from fat) will help you manage your weight and reduce your risk for disease, such as heart disease, high blood pressure, and cancer. Don't forget, though, that the total calories you eat are still an important part of managing your weight.

- Save high-fat foods for a special occasion. Fat is a concentrated source of calories, and it is tasty, making it easy to eat too many calories. Use the tips for cutting fat and choosing lean meats and meat alternatives to help you decrease some high-fat foods in your diet.

- Limit liquids and foods that are high in sugar. Beverages and foods that contain sugar add calories but may not add much nutrition to your diet. Substitute water for high-sugar drinks (including high-sugar juice drinks). Don't substitute diet drinks, which contain higher levels of sodium and caffeine.

- Eat plenty of foods high in iron and calcium. If you are a woman of childbearing age, be sure you get plenty of folic acid in your diet to reduce your chances of having a child with birth defects.

- If you drink alcohol, drink moderate amounts (no more than two drinks a day for a man or one drink a day for a woman). Drinking excess alcohol increases abdominal fat, increasing your risk for heart disease and Type 2 diabetes.

WEIGH YOURSELF LESS OFTEN

Your weight can fluctuate by a few pounds from one day to another. However, over the long run, most people's weight stays fairly stable. The fluctuations you see from day to day are changes in the amount of water in your body. The adult body is about 60 percent water, so small changes in water balance can easily alter body weight. For example, it is normal for many women to have some water retention around the time of their menstrual period, so their weight increases temporarily by a few pounds during this time.

What you eat can also influence how much water your body retains. If you eat a very salty meal, your body will retain extra water for one or two days to keep your body fluids from being too salty. Afterward, your body will get rid of both the extra salt and water through your urine.

Because of daily fluctuations in your weight, you should not weigh yourself every day. Instead of weighing, you can rely on how you feel and how your clothes fit. If you want to monitor your weight, you should weigh yourself no more than once a week (unless directed by your doctor to weigh yourself more often because of a health concern).

CHANGE FOR LIFE

If weight loss is one of your goals to improve your health, it is not necessary to lose all your excess weight to improve it. Research shows that improvements in health can be achieved by losing as little as 5 to 10 percent of your weight. A reasonable time to plan for losing 10 percent is six months.

- If your Body Mass Index (BMI) is between twenty-seven and thirty-five you can reduce your caloric intake by three hundred to five hundred calories a day and lose 0.5 to 1 pound a week, for a 10 percent weight loss in six months.

Losing weight slowly will help keep the weight off in the long run. After six months of weight loss, you will likely find that losing additional weight is not as easy. This is because your body has adjusted to the new weight and is conserving more energy. You will need to continue your weight-management program or you will gain the weight back. If you need to lose more weight, your total daily calories will need to be reduced more and your physical activity increased.

Follow the ABCs (Aim for fitness, Build a healthy base, and Choose sensibly) to reach your healthy weight and improve your health. Believe in your ability to change and keep reminding yourself of your new health goals. Monitor the changes you are making in your life.

Here are some additional tips to help you be successful in making and maintaining changes that you can follow for the rest of your life.

- Manage stress.

- Manage your environment.

- Prevent relapse.

- Get support from a variety of sources. There are books, support groups, seminars, and trusted friends and relatives. You may also find it helpful to seek professional counseling—especially if you think you have emotional issues or may be depressed. A registered dietitian can help you learn more about the Food Guide Pyramid and setting up a healthy food plan for yourself.

- Reward yourself for small accomplishments rather than waiting until you have completely reached your goal. Treat yourself to a movie, new CD, an afternoon off work, or an hour of quiet time. Rewarding yourself for small achievements along the way will help keep you focused on your goals.

THE WAY OBESITY IS MEASURED CAN BE MISLEADING

It is well documented that being overweight or obese is associated with numerous serious health risks. However, researchers have been finding that people can be healthy, fit, and fat. In 1998, the National Heart, Lung, and Blood Institute (NHLBI) released the first federal guidelines on identifying, evaluating, and treating overweight and obesity in adults. These guidelines lowered the thresholds for being obese and overweight, instantly putting many more people in these categories. The institute defined being overweight as having a Body Mass Index (BMI) of 25 to 29.9 and being obese as having a BMI of 30 or above. BMI is calculated as weight in kilograms divided by height in meters squared.)

Using BMI as an obesity measurement has its limitations. BMI is not a reliable predictor of fitness level or blood pressure and does not distinguish between lean and fat tissue (the single most important factor in determining obesity). Moreover, BMI does not take into account race, ethnicity, age, or gender. For these reasons, some researchers have warned that using BMI as the sole measurement of healthy weight may do more harm than good.

RESEARCH SAYS YOU *CAN* BE FIT AND FAT

To the question "Can a person be healthy and fat?" an increasing number of experts are answering, "Yes!"

Researchers examined 21,925 men of all shapes and sizes. The investigators assessed the men's body composition and then closely monitored their medical histories for an average of eight years. They found that the men who were fat and fit did not have an elevated mortality rate. In fact, the fat, fit men had a lower mortality rate than the normal weight men who were unfit. Other studies have confirmed that low fitness, caused by being sedentary, is more important than obesity as an indicator of mortality and that poor cardiorespiratory fitness is a strong, independent predictor of death by any cause (Lee, Blair, and Jackson, 1999, *Journal of the American Medical Association* 69, no. 3).

DOCTORS OFTEN FAIL TO EMPHASIZE EXERCISE

Using indicators like BMI, medical professionals continue to focus on weight loss alone, neglecting exercise. Yet exercise can result in substantial levels of aerobic fitness, flexibility, muscular strength, and endurance.

LOSING WEIGHT ISN'T ALWAYS THE ANSWER

There is no doubt that weight loss can benefit the health of many people who are defined as obese or overweight, particularly if the weight is lost by making permanent lifestyle changes, such as adhering to a healthier diet and participating in regular exercise. However, the reality is that losing weight is daunting to those who have constantly struggled with their weight.

FIT AND FAT ROLE MODELS SHOW THE WAY

An increasing number of people are living proof that it is possible to be fit and fat. Take Joe Athlete, for example. At five feet, eight inches tall, he weighs 250 pounds, has a BMI of thirty-eight, and is considered morbidly obese. He has also completed 264 triathlons. A typical training week consists of swimming five miles, running thirty, and cycling two hundred. He has a resting pulse of sixty beats per minute, his blood pressure is 120 over 80, and he has perfectly normal stress-level results. In short, he is a fit, healthy athlete.

THE TRUTH ABOUT STEROIDS

Steroid abuse is still on the rise, and not just among professional athletes and bodybuilders. Despite numerous educational efforts by health care officials, many amateur and high school athletes looking for that elusive competitive edge still believe they can get it from a syringe or a bottle of pills. What they don't realize is that steroids will give them a lot more than they bargained for.

NOT WORTH THE RISK

Acne, liver damage, increased risk of heart disease, these are just a few of the side effects associated with anabolic steroid abuse. And there's more.

The side effects are severe. Men who use steroids also may develop gynecomastia (the development of breasts), priapism (painful prolonged erection), and edema from sodium and water retention. They also will be more prone to cardiovascular problems since steroids decrease high-density lipoprotein levels (HDL) or "good" cholesterol and increase low-density lipoprotein levels (LDL) or "bad" cholesterol. Coupled with hypertension and negative changes in myocardial tissue, steroid users are at an increased risk for heart attacks as well.

Of additional concern are alterations in psyche and behavior (i.e., aggression, physical dependence) and decreased immune function. Changes in the reproductive system, such as a reduction in testicle size, sperm count, and mobility, and a decrease in the levels of endogenous testosterone and other sex hormones are common.

ALL RISK, NO GLORY

There is an even scarier risk of steroid abuse: death. Steroid users who share needles are putting themselves at risk for developing infections such as HIV, hepatitis, or other viral diseases.

The terminal risks of steroid abuse are not fully known. Some published cases of tumors and other cancers related to steroid abuse have been reported. Even so, physicians and researchers do not know all the repercussions of steroid abuse on one's body and future health. Controlled research is unethical, and only information from abusers is usable; yet this data may be inaccurate since most users are not forthcoming about the full extent of their steroid use.

Since the late 1980s, the federal government has begun to crack down on steroid use and distribution. Possession of steroids with intent to distribute without a valid prescription is a felony and subject to prosecution. Likewise, steroid use is a violation of the rules of virtually all sports leagues and councils as well as the traditional ethics of good sportsmanship.

NO SUBSTITUTE FOR TRAINING

What most steroid users don't realize is that they are placing themselves at risk for something they could achieve on their own. Many experts agree that the effects of steroids on strength and muscle mass of beginning weight lifters or athletes are minimal when compared with the effects of an intensive weight-training or conditioning program.

The best way to improve performance and increase muscle mass is to follow a well-designed program that challenges both your body and your mind. No drug can do that for you.

CREATINE CREATES A SENSATION

Even if you don't know exactly what it is, chances are you've probably heard about creatine. With help from the media and high-profile athletes, this popular supplement exploded onto the scene several years ago as news spread of its potential as a muscle builder and sports-performance enhancer. As further proof of its popularity, sales of creatine have skyrocketed from $30 million in 1995 to a projected $180 million in 1998.

Perhaps the greatest testament to creatine's effectiveness and, hence, its popularity is the fact that so many who use it are professional and amateur athletes alike, who actually see results, fast results. Unlike predecessors such as chromium picolinate, creatine has, from the outset, consistently demonstrated its usefulness in a variety of applications in numerous scientific studies. More than fifty studies examining creatine have been published and another fifty are expected to be published before year's end.

But neither its popularity nor reports of its effectiveness have completely erased the doubt and fears of those who question the safety of creatine supplementation. A recent survey of the Association of Professional Team Physicians indicated 85 percent would not recommend creatine until more research was completed. And because no study of creatine has lasted longer than fifty-one days, it is impossible to know its long-term effects.

WHO IS IT FOR?

Each of us has varying levels of creatine stored in our muscles depending on our diets, activity levels, and genetics. Those who appear to benefit most from creatine supplementation are those with the lowest amounts to begin with. After the initial recommended loading phase of twenty to twenty-five grams per day for five to seven days, the muscles becomes saturated with creatine and additional supplementation beyond a three- to five-gram maintenance dose becomes a wasted and expensive enterprise. In fact, the daily turnover rate for creatine is only about two grams per day, making large doses not only unnecessary, but potentially harmful since protocols deviating from the recommended dosages have yet to be studied.

The sports performance benefits of creatine are limited to activities requiring short, all-out bursts of power, such as:

- Jumping

- Swimming

- Sprinting

- High-intensity weight lifting

A recent statement by the American College of Sports Medicine (ACSM) notes that "creatine supplementation has not been shown to improve longer-duration aerobic-type exercise."

THE "MORE IS BETTER" SYNDROME

The controversy that continues to hound creatine stems from the fact that the controlled setting of a lab does not always reflect real life. In a if-a-little-is-good-more-is-better society like ours, it's no surprise that many people are taking far more than the recommended dosage of creatine, which is something the researchers have yet to examine. And few studies have been able to demonstrate creatine's effectiveness beyond the lab setting on a baseball field, for example, or at a track meet.

"Much remains unknown about whether creatine is absolutely safe for long-term use at levels currently being recommended," said the Food and Drug Administration (FDA) in a June 1998 statement cautioning consumers about the popular supplement. The FDA urges both current and potential users to see their doctors to identify any potential health problems. Creatine supplementation is not for everyone, particularly those with a history of kidney problems or who are younger than age eighteen or who are still developing. Nor should one expect the supplement to be effective without a well-designed training program. Every person should examine their own motives for taking creatine and weigh them against the potential unknown risks of long-term usage. But be sure to take the FDA's advice and check with your physician and don't exceed the recommended dose.

HOW IT WORKS

Here's how researchers believe creatine works: In its phosphorylated form, creatine plays a key role in the formation of ATP, the body's energy source. Without enough creatine, which is created in the liver and kidneys and stored in the muscle, the cycle that creates this energy is unable to produce enough ATP to meet the demands of short bursts of muscle activity. Researchers have discovered that a shortage of creatine can cause muscle fatigue. Because it is a nonanabolic substance naturally found in the body, researchers believe creatine to be a safer alternative to other muscle-enhancing drugs or potions.

IF YOU DON'T USE IT, WILL YOU LOSE IT?

If you've been sidelined by an injury or you're considering taking a break from exercise, you might wonder if you'll lose your hard-earned strength and endurance. Some loss of fitness is inevitable, but there are ways to help minimize it. Here's what happens to your body when you take a break from exercise.

MATTERS OF THE HEART

The degree to which cardiovascular fitness declines during a period of detraining depends upon what kind of shape you were in to begin with. Individuals who are extremely fit, such as highly trained athletes, experience a rapid drop in fitness during the first three weeks of detraining, which then tapers off. A significant level of fitness—higher than that of an untrained person—is retained for about twelve weeks. Individuals with low-to-moderate fitness levels show little change in cardiovascular fitness within the first few weeks, but their ability rapidly declines in the weeks immediately following.

PERFORMANCE JITTERS

The ability to perform a given sport or activity, whether it involves swinging a bat in softball or run-

ning ten kilometers, invariably declines when the sport is abandoned for any length of time. One study found that marathoners experienced a 25 percent decrease in endurance time during a maximal aerobic treadmill test after just fifteen days of inactivity. Another showed that a swimmers' arm strength declined by more than 13 percent within four weeks of abandoning their regular training regimen.

Numerous variables come into play when analyzing the ability to perform a particular sport-specific skill, making it difficult to analyze the effects of detraining. Some are like riding a bike—you never forget how—while others, such as the ability to deliver an accurate serve in tennis, for example, involve specific timing and well-trained muscles.

SPEAKING OF MUSCLES . . .

With the exception of a genetically blessed few, most of us have to work at it, building strength through formal or informal strength-training workouts. Again, well-trained athletes have the edge because the positive effects of training remain evident weeks, sometimes even months, after ending training. Lesser trained individuals can expect to see their muscle strength and conditioning decline at a slightly faster rate, though not at the levels seen in sedentary individuals.

STEM THE DETRAINING TIDE

Experts agree that the best way to avoid losing much of the health and fitness benefits you've worked so hard to achieve is to do something. If you can't find the motivation to run for a few weeks or longer, try walking instead. Crosstraining became popular because it is a viable means of maintaining, even increasing, one's fitness level. Runners can give their knees a break by switching to cycling, swimmers can work their legs on a stair stepper, and aerobics enthusiasts can take their workout outdoors by hiking through a local park or reserve.

If an injury is keeping you from your favorite activities, take your worries to the pool. Of course, it's always advisable to check with your physician before resuming exercise after an injury. Regardless of which activity you choose, be sure to progress gradually.

If boredom is the problem, now's the time to try that sport you've been considering for so long. In-line skating, tai chi, boot-camp workouts—whatever strikes your fancy. The key is to keep your heart and muscles challenged in order to minimize the detraining effects that come when taking a break from your usual routine.

CHAPTER TEN

STRESS AND DESTRESSING

Stress is and will forever be a part of our world. Think of it: traffic, long lines, noise, media, health concerns, family responsibilities, money, deadlines, the chaos of the world. This is our world. Unless you decide to move to the mountaintops of Colorado or join an Amish group in Pennsylvania, you will have a hard time avoiding stress. If you can't avoid it, then you have to do something about it. You need to learn how to relax and invite a downtime period to your day.

Stress is a natural response to stimuli. It is that simple. The environment and society contribute to the stress that our bodies deal with. As the outside world challenges us, the internal systems of the body react and allow us to adapt to those changes and survive. Take, for example, reading this book, completely absorbed by the words of wisdom I am giving you when you hear a loud crash outside your door. Your senses become alert, and your body is at attention. Where did that come from? Who is it? What was that? Am I in danger? Your muscles tense up and your heart is pounding faster and you may break into a little sweat. You try to quiet your throbbing heart and slow down your breathing, prying your fingers away from the edge of this book. Your instincts are telling you to fight, run, or hide. This is your body reacting naturally to stress. It will want to fight or run naturally.

The same response can help you in meeting goals and day-to-day challenges that require you to reach your peak performance ability. In this respect stress can work for you instead of against you. Stress becomes a problem when unrelieved or chronic. Your body is in a constant state of alertness, and the protective responses that your body deals with naturally make you feel sick. This is a harmful effect on your mental and physical well-being that too much stress can create.

What happens in your body when stress messages are received? It is like beaming information from a Palm Pilot, the information goes in, but the body has to find a way to process the information. There are some physiological changes that will occur:

1. Heart rate and blood pressure increase.

2. Oxygen consumption rises and your respiratory rate goes up.

3. Adrenaline, hormones, and fatty acids are released into the bloodstream.

4. Muscles tense.

5. Liver releases sugar.

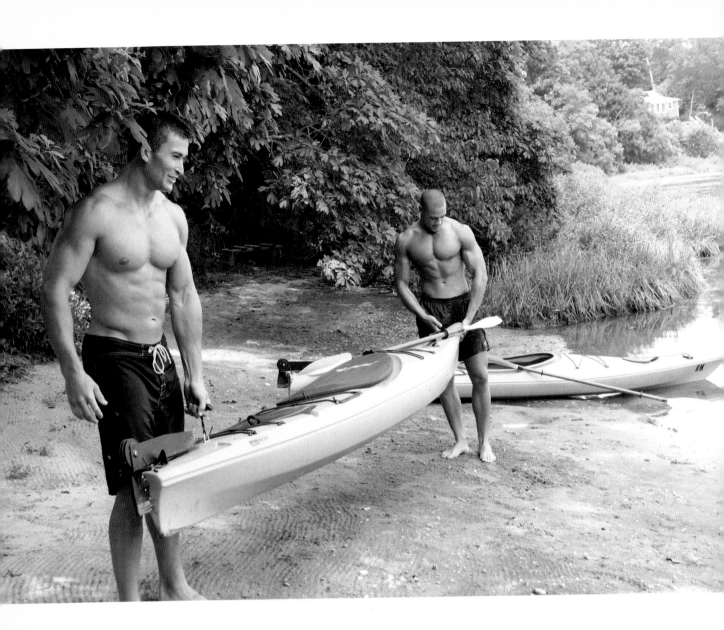

6. Blood flow to the digestive organs and extremities is constricted.

7. Blood flow to the brain and major muscles increases.

8. Metabolism increases, creating heat so the body perspires to cool itself.

LONG-TERM EFFECTS

This is an everyday ordeal that the body has to endure. There are most likely twenty-five to thirty minor stresses that happen each and every day. Although many of them are minor, they are relentless. Other stress are not so minor—worrying about your job, illness, or the health of someone close to you; the state of the world, as we know it; a bad breakup. This type of stressful stimulus lingers for long periods of time. When all that stress builds up, your body and emotions feel the strain. Eventually the load becomes too great to bear. The brain will have too many things to worry about, so even the most insignificant thing will cause a big physical reaction.

Doctors have recognized a direct link between

stress and some of our most common ailments and disorders, such as asthma, intestinal problems, heart disease, and other respiratory conditions that can aggravate us. Headaches and migraines can be brought on or even worsened by stress. Emotional problems like depression and anxiety are frequently stress related as well.

There is strong evidence that chronic stress breaks down the immune system, increasing your chances of getting sick. The constant presence of stress hormones in the bloodstream blocks the body's defense systems (lymphocytes), weakening the ability to combat disease.

HOW DO YOU SPELL RELIEF? EXERCISE

Exercise in many forms helps to relieve physical symptoms of stress. Aerobic movement, flexibility training, weight training, and coordination skills will help destress you in several ways. Here are a few.

1. Moving will help relax tense muscle.

2. During an exercise period your body will produce chemicals that calm the stress response and offer a calming or euphoric state.

3. Exercise utilizes excess hormones, fatty acids, and sugar, which are elevated in the bloodstream due to stress.

4. Exercisers and sports enthusiasts are better able to relax and can relax under pressure easier.

5. That euphoric state gained from exercise lasts for hours after training.

Taking small steps to include physical activity that will reduce stress can be as easy as taking a fifteen-minute walk during lunch, walking to and from work if possible, even stretching out your back and shoulders at your desk can offer some relief. It doesn't have to involve a gym membership and clothes to change into, scheduling a date and time, and other variables that will only counteract the reason you are doing this in the first place. Another helpful hint would be to reduce some of the caffeine and sugar that stimulates you into hyperdrive. It may be as simple as getting some air and taking your mind off things for a few minutes instead of fueling the tiger in your head.

THE GOOD, THE BAD, AND THE UGLY

Good stresses can help us control bad stresses. Playing a tennis match, shooting baskets, or even lifting weights can help your body react to stress through mastery of the task at hand. Your heart rate elevates, your brain strategizes and problem solves, and your muscles are working. Your body and mind work together to win. Once you recognize how the mind and body work together as a team, the easier it will become for you to manage everyday stress.

Where does the ugly come in? Stress can also produce a scowl on your face. The weight of the world weighs down your body and puts worry lines on your face. Athletes and active people shine with enthusiasm and burst with the kinds of vitality I wish I could package. That kind of positive energy comes from within, but so does negative stress. Once you feel what athletes feel, you won't go back.

How you react to stressful situations will determine how your body copes with stress. Some people find new situations to be interesting challenges and some find new situations uncomfortable and stressful challenges. A positive response of this formula means you can overcome the stress and work it out internally to meet the challenge. A negative response makes you feel "out of control" and doubtful. Exercise will be your ally and give you a better sense of control and self-confidence to enable you to cope with everyday stresses.

Physical training and the stamina and courage you'll gain through exercise will trickle over into almost every part of your life. Don't forget that enjoyment is a vital stress reliever. Find a way to relax and give yourself over to your chosen program. Approach each session with attainable goals and expectations. Instead of considering working out a chore, look at it as a way of taking care of you. Instead of worrying about beating the other guy, think of the competition as being with your own body and mind.

STRESS BUSTERS

REKINDLE AN OLD PASSION

Think of something you used to do in college or high school that gave you pleasure. What did you do in your spare time that you don't have time to do anymore? Painting, reading, riding a bike, playing a musical instrument, day trips, hiking, or camping? These are many activities that we use to enjoy but that we seem to discount as adults. Look back to these activities to provide you time and space from the familiar grind. These activities are often things we truly loved to do as kids, and they can have huge value revisited as adults. Some men have the opportunity to join group activities through sports or even health clubs or private clubs. Even shooting hoops with the guys over the weekend can give you a boost. Try to invest in activities that help you remember what life was like when the only care in the world was the moment you were

in. Try to find that passion and you will find yourself.

GET A PET—ANY SHAPE OR SIZE WILL DO

The best idea I've had to take down my stress level and change my attitude was getting a dog. At first it seemed as though the additional responsibility would be overwhelming. Anyone who owns a pet will tell you that your focus shifts when that new addition walks, crawls, swims, or flies its way into your life. Suddenly the spotlight shines less on you and the problems of the day, but on this creature that only wags its tail, licks your face, and loves you no matter what. Studies have shown that pets of almost any kind provide calming physical effects.

MEDITATE NOT *MEDICATE*

If your life can resemble a hurricane, think of meditating as the eye of the storm, a place to find refuge.

WHAT IS MEDITATION? Meditation has been practiced in many cultures throughout the ages and is not necessarily a religious activity. With practice, you can learn how to move into a serene state of mind. The goal is to achieve "pure awareness" or complete consciousness. Scientists, spiritual leaders, philosophers, and psychologists have spent lifetimes trying to define this apparently simple concept. The term most frequently used to describe our "being" is *spirit*. Spirit is defined as the animating force of life. Many great teachers throughout the ages have said that spirit can be found in the space *between* our thoughts. To find this place, we must slow down and look inward.

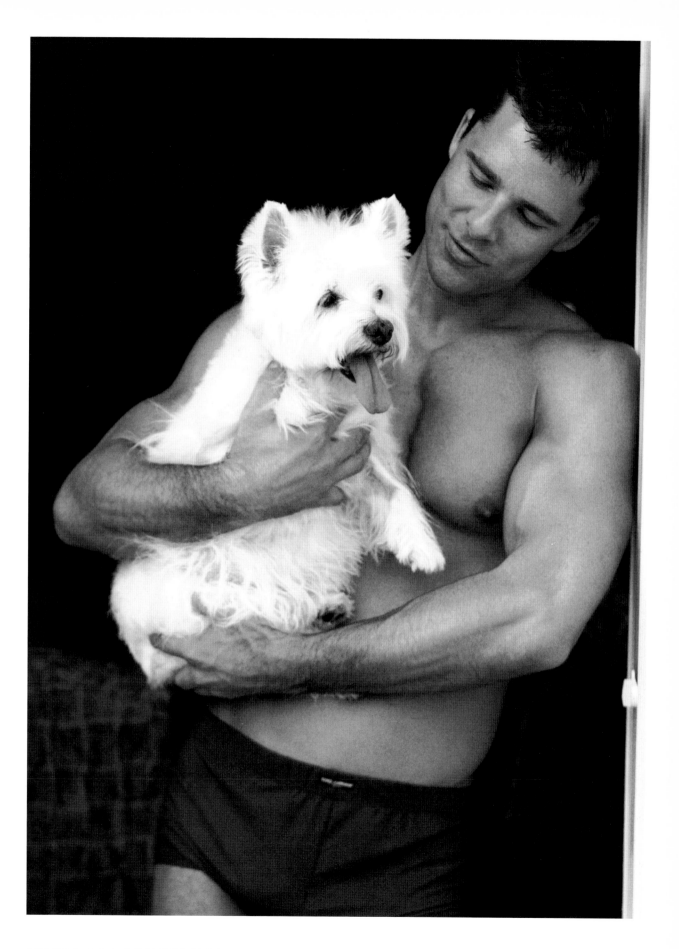

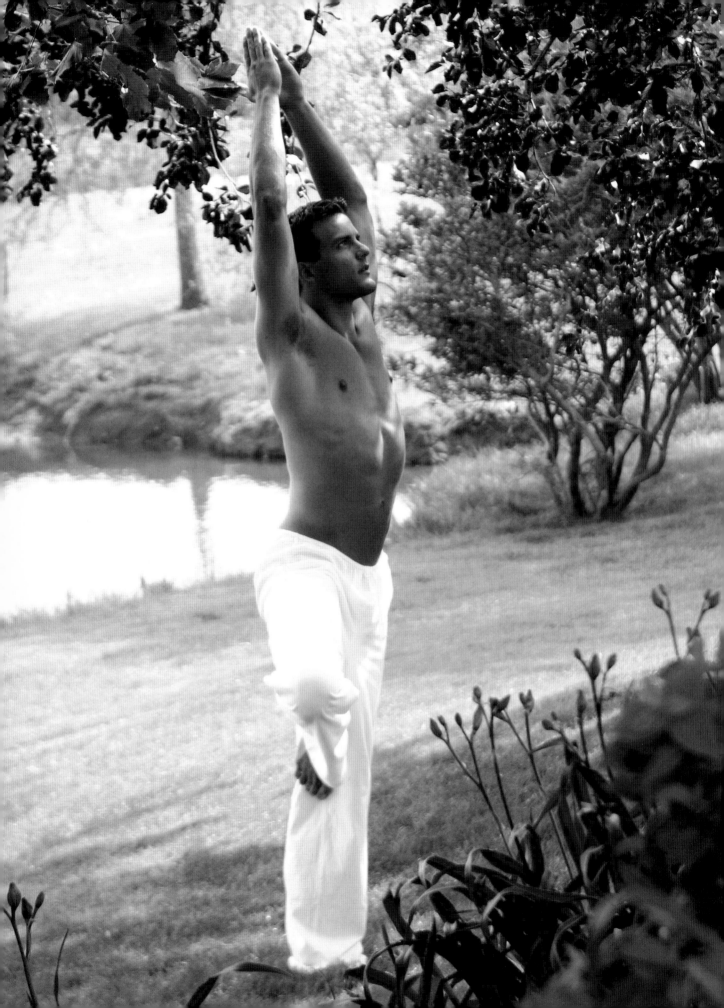

LOOKING INWARD. The challenge of looking inward or moving into "pure awareness" is to let go of any attachment to specific thoughts. Our mind seems to conduct a one-way conversation with itself. Most often our thoughts are focused on the past or the future.

We rarely live in the richness and fullness of the present moment. The present moment is what is real; being fully aware and engaged in it is the goal most of us want to achieve through meditation.

PRACTICING MEDITATION. There are many variations of meditation techniques; those taught in specific yoga practices, those taught by fellowships or by spiritual leaders, health care groups, stress-reduction groups, and those that are self-taught. Three practices commonly used in the West include:

- *Concentration on an object.*

- *Watching the breath.*

- *Reciting a mantra.*

OBJECT CONCENTRATION. Focus your gaze on a single object. An inspirational object, like a flower or stream, is most helpful. Many gaze lightly into the flame of a candle. The goal is to bring the mind to one point of focus in the present moment.

WATCHING THE BREATH. Also referred to as mindfulness meditation. Observe your breath while sitting quietly. Thoughts will move through your mind, but keep your attention on your breath. Follow your breath as it flows in and out of your lungs. Notice the space between the "in and out" breaths. If your mind wanders—and it most likely will—simply bring it back to the breath. Watching the breath helps you realize that you are not the collection of your thoughts, but a being that goes beyond your thoughts.

MANTRA MEDITATION. *Mantra* means "control of mind." In mantra meditation you repeat a word or series of words to help you gain control of a restless mind. The mantra doesn't have to be foreign to you. Simple yet powerful words—like "joy, peace, bliss" or "peace, harmony, and well-being"—are very effective.

To realize the benefits of meditation, a regular practice is required. Just as you train your body through a consistent program of exercise, in meditation you train your mind through consistent practice. You'll open up to new levels of mental clarity, physical health, and spiritual inspiration.

BRAIN TRAINING

For some time there has been compelling evidence to show that exercise helps elevate brain function. Recent research has begun to quantify the parts of the brain that are actually stimulated by particular types of exercise. One of the most interesting findings is that the type of exercise you do can have a direct or indirect impact on the cerebellum. The cerebellum's main function is to control and coordinate muscular activity and maintain balance. Exercises that use the lower body, specifically the legs, and incorporate balance, strength, and dexterity help exercise the brain's balance and coordination centers. The added benefit, of course, is that you can increase strength and sports performance with lower body work. Here are some simple activities that will strengthen the link between the body and the brain:

Engage in gentle Eastern-based disciplines such as yoga, tai chi, and some Pilates movements. Concentrating on slow, correct movement is important in these activities. The goal is to create balance and stillness. It is not necessary to dive into a class or perform sixty minutes of a particular discipline. Even five minutes, using a few specific movements two times a week, can have an effect.

Use stability and medicine balls to perform exercises that utilize your body weight and require you to stabilize yourself with one or both legs and/or your torso while performing them. Slow down your movements and hold positions for several seconds to force yourself to engage your cerebellum as well as your muscle groups.

Use a stationary cycle or elliptical trainer in ways that promote balance and coordination. Try single-leg pedaling for short periods of time. Slightly lift one foot from the platform and perform your elliptical trainer routine with most of your weight on the other foot for short periods. Walk on your treadmill with a slow, lunging motion that requires you to work much harder on your balance. Perform very light dumbbell-resistance exercises while balancing on one leg. Concentrate on simple lifts, where your arms do not go above your shoulders, e.g., dumbbell curls. Try standing on a balance or wobble board. Practice balance by walking the length of your driveway on a narrow curb, pausing from time to time to balance on one leg.

These exercises can be done at the beginning or end of your regular strength, flexibility, or aerobic routine. Many of my clients over the years have found that adding balance and coordination movements to their routine helps them play their sports or pursue other recreational activities at a higher level. This includes golf, tennis, snowboarding, mountain climbing, and basketball. Remember that the goal of these types of exercises is to stimulate the cerebellum and add dimension to your routine to promote physical well-roundedness.

Some of these exercises can be challenging, particularly those that utilize weights or balls. Make sure that you get the proper guidance from a certified fitness professional on form, the amount of weight, and the number of repetitions before you include these in your routine. One-legged exercises can also put added stress on your knees and ankle joints, so make sure that you are cleared by your physician before exercising if you have preexisting medical conditions in these areas.

TEN THINGS YOU CAN DO RIGHT NOW TO LOOK GREAT LATER; TEN ACTIONS THAT YOU SHOULD MAKE HABIT FORMING.

1. GIVE UP ONE FOOD ITEM THAT YOU OVERINDULGE IN. I gave up french fries and reduced my body fat by 2 percent. I don't think that it was just the fries, it was the foods that I ate with the fries on the side. You pay more attention to your diet when you impose a small restriction on food choices. And adjustment makes it tougher to eat thoughtlessly. Try it for just a short time and see if you notice a difference.

2. CHANGE YOUR AEROBIC ACTIVITY DRASTICALLY. You may be coasting along, your cardio training on autopilot. Your body needs a shake up to strip it of unwanted fat. Try changing your routine cardio session to one that is completely different in every way. Your body will go into overdrive to relearn how to use energy (fat), and therefore you will burn more of the lard than you did before. You might consider trying a spinning (indoor cycle) class at your club. There are many studios that allow you to take individual classes so you can try something new. This will definitely kick you into overdrive!

3. INTENSIFY YOUR CURRENT PROGRAM. Many of us

have a set level of intensity that we feel comfortable with and accept a predictable set of results after every workout. If you challenge yourself by hiking up the intensity levels on a gradual scale, your body will respond by working harder and creating results faster.

4. JUMP ROPE. Pull out a skill that you most likely haven't used since high school. You will be amazed at how efficient jumping rope is and how intense the training can be. Learn proper techniques by video or just get a rope and start. Some tips. Don't jump too high in the air, about three inches off the ground is enough for each rotation. Keep your hands down along the sides of your hips when you jump and rotate from the forearm rather than the wrist. Try jumping for fifty rotations at first and build your endurance; you should shoot for about five or ten minutes. Jumping rope is incredibly efficient: you should see results after about three weeks if you jump three to four times a week.

5. CHANGE THE TIME YOU HIT THE GYM. Not only is there an entire "new" group of men in the gym to inspire you, but you may find that your focus is different if you go in before work or make time to work the day's frustrations off in the evening.

6. TEST DRIVE A HOME WORK-OUT VIDEO. Sometimes it takes trying something at home for you to feel comfortable enough doing it to start a new program. There's a huge array of tapes out there for you to choose from, covering everything from Tae Bo to nude yoga. Rent from an Internet site or catalog to find tapes that really inspire you before you invest in a purchase.

7. TRY A MARTIAL ARTS CLASS. Kickboxing classes and other combative forms of exercise are now widely available in gyms and clubs around America. These classes are often very effective if taught by an expert, but I believe you would be better off finding a true martial

arts course (karate, tae kwon do) taught by a sensei with years of experience and leadership. Most martial arts are more than just kicking and punching; they are ways of life.

8. TAKE THE STAIRS. Use stairs as an alternative to the elevator and give those hidden bursts of energy an outlet that can really make a difference in your body-fat ratio. It seems like a baby step, but most major health organizations in America suggest that accumulative aerobic activity for just twenty minutes a day will have an effect on your body and help you lose weight. You won't lose ten pounds by the fifth floor, but you will boost your heart rate a bit and tone your leg muscles. Don't be as quick to take the stairs down, however. Going down stairs may cause undue impact to the knee joint.

9. TRY WEARING A HEART-RATE MONITOR WHEN YOU TRAIN. If you understand the concept of heart-rate monitoring, you will train more efficiently and achieve visible results much faster, with more or less output. Monitoring is like driving with a map. It helps you understand how hard to push and where you are at any given moment of a workout. You may also enjoy using a techy toy to get into shape.

10. INTERNET SUPPORT. Now there are many Web sites (including my own, JonGiswold.com) set up to help you develop a balanced training plan. These sites give you information about nutrition, offer support, and feature chat rooms with other men and women who share your goals. They also spotlight new products, new trends, and cutting-edge research. You can even connect through your PDA.

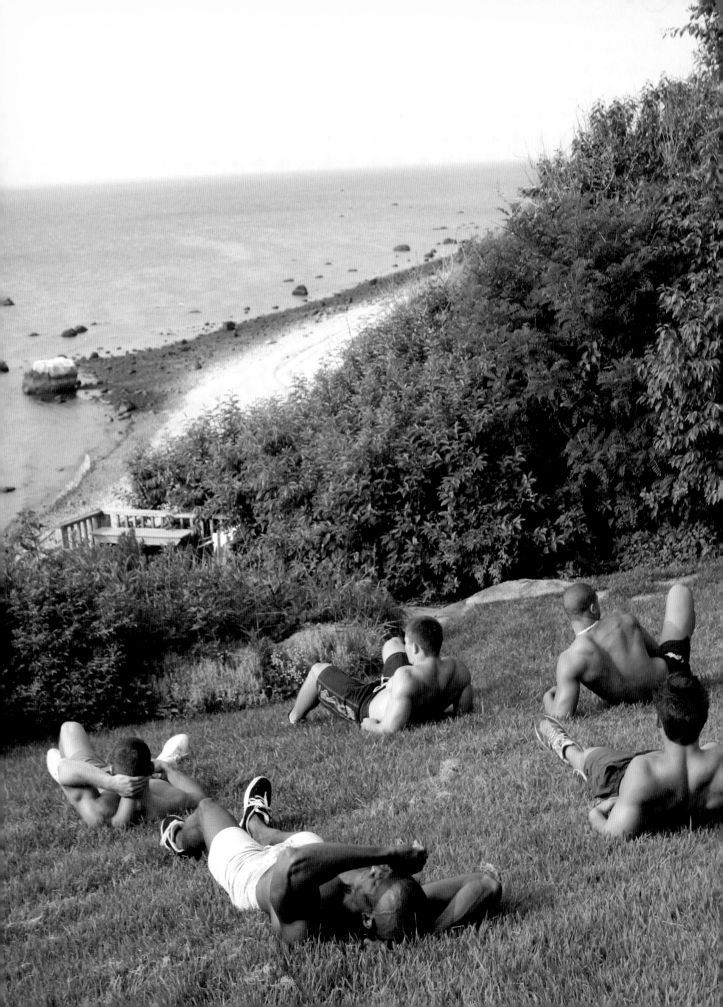

CHAPTER ELEVEN

BEYOND EXERCISE

Whether you want to begin exercising as a result of your physician's recommendation or your own initiative, talk with your practitioner before you start. Ask for specific programming recommendations. Many physicians or physical therapists provide instructions for exercises unique to specific conditions (i.e., back exercises for low-back pain). Inquire about special limitations of which you should be aware, and ask your physician if they can refer you to a fitness professional who has experience training clients with your condition.

CERTIFIED FITNESS PROFESSIONALS MAKE A DIFFERENCE

You may benefit from working with a certified fitness professional. Communication is important. Do they have experience working with your condition? Would they feel comfortable training you? If not, could they refer you to someone with experience? Do they provide knowledgeable answers to your questions? Don't hesitate to ask what you can expect to achieve with an exercise program and be sure to discuss your goals.

Expect to tell the fitness professional about your general health, any specific illness or injury, and your physical-activity history. They may perform evaluations, such as a range-of-motion test for a certain joint or cardiorespiratory testing to measure heart rate during aerobic exercise. The fitness professional will use this information to establish realistic goals and design a safe, effective exercise program. If you feel the fitness professional does not seem familiar with your condition, find another professional who is.

SOMETIMES HEALTH AND FITNESS PROFESSIONALS NEED TO TALK

Your fitness trainer may feel it's necessary to speak with your health-care professional before working with you. The trainer or instructor may require specific guidance on a safe range of motion for your joints or a proper approach if you have risk factors for heart disease. The fitness professional also may need to clarify physical-activity program goals even if a physician referred you. These discussions may take time, but be patient—thoroughness is in your best interest.

PROGRESSION

Regardless of whether you exercise in a group or one-on-one, training should progress from an initial, easy effort level to one that's more challenging. A group instructor should provide modifications, if necessary, specific to your condition. A personal trainer also should offer exercises performed at appropriate ranges of motion and intensities. Both types of fitness professionals should be able to explain why they recommend certain exercises and provide you with a plan that details the progress you can expect.

Exercise can be an important, fulfilling part of coping with a chronic disease or recovering from an injury. Coordinate with your health-care provider and fitness professional to make the most of your exercise experience and to improve your ability to function throughout your life.

EXERCISING WITH A HEALTH CHALLENGE

People facing various health challenges are not precluded from the benefits of exercise. In fact, physical activity can help increase energy, strength, balance, and coordination, as well as ease pain.

INJURIES

The anterior cruciate ligament, or ACL, is a cord inside the knee that helps stabilize the knee joint. It is one of the most commonly injured ligaments in the knee, especially in sports that involve direct contact to the joint, as well as jumping, running, and twisting of the knee, such as football. Typically, the knee gives with a popping sound and swells up. If the ACL ruptures or suffers a large tear, most professional players elect to get it surgically replaced by a graft. It usually takes four months or more to recover from the injury.

A sprain refers to a torn or stretched ligament—the body's connectors that join different bones together in a joint. Ankle sprains, possibly the most common athletic injury, usually happen to a ligament on the outer side of the ankle (the side of the little toe) and may involve just a stretch, a partial tear, or a complete tear. They usually are very painful and cause the ankle to swell. Though the diagnosis can be made just by questioning the player and examining the ankle, doctors usually take an X ray to check for other damage. RICE (which stands for rest, ice, compression, and elevation) is the standard treatment. Surgery may be needed for extreme tears or repeated tears to repair or replace the ligament. Most players recover in three to six weeks. Taping the ankle, wearing high-top athletic shoes, stretching, and strengthening can help prevent the injury.

A concussion is a brain injury caused by a sharp blow to the head. It can hurt the brain at the site of the blow or can cause the brain to jolt away from the blow and hit the inside of the skull. The player can be confused or dizzy and, in severe cases, may lose consciousness. Treatment ranges from simple pain killers and overnight monitoring (in which the player is awakened every few hours to make sure there are no brain symptoms) to CT scans, MRIs, and X rays to detect whether there is any damage to the brain, skull, or spine. Players also might get a silent injury, in which a small artery bleeds into the skull, and the effects are not apparent for several hours. Helmets and proper football techniques are the best ways to prevent this injury.

The ligaments, muscles, and capsules in the shoulder help keep the bones together to form the shoulder while allowing it to be an extremely mobile joint. A dislocated shoulder occurs when the ball-like upper end of the arm bone separates from its socket. Doctors usually can diagnose the condition by a clinical exam, but sometimes an X ray may be called for. A doctor can perform a simple maneuver to reset the joint, after which strengthening exercises and physical therapy help rehabilitate it. In severe or recurrent cases, doctors may either use heat probes to shrink the capsule or surgically correct the problem.

The medial collateral ligament, or MCL, is a ligament inside the knee that helps stabilize the knee joint. It typically suffers direct traumatic injury from the outer side of the knee, which routinely injures the ACL as well. Typically, the knee gives with a popping sound and swells up. An MCL injury is usually treated with RICE (rest, ice, compression, and elevation), as well as physical therapy and pain medications. The joint may be immobilized but usually is not put in a cast.

In healthy shoulder ligaments, muscles and other structures hold the arm, the collarbone, and the shoulder blade together to form the shoulder joint. In a separated shoulder, most often the ligaments holding the collarbone in place tear and cause the collarbone to pop up. This should not be confused with a dislocated shoulder, in which the arm bone comes out of its socket, or a rotator cuff injury, in which a group of muscles holding the shoulder together gets partially or completely torn. A clinical exam and X ray usually are all that is needed to make the diagnosis of a separated shoulder. Wearing an arm sling, compressing with ice, and receiving physical therapy are the usual components of treatment. In football, the injury usually is caused by the player slamming into a hard object, such as the turf. Here correct padding is the best prevention.

A stinger usually happens when a football player lands on his head and shoulder (or collides with another player in the same way). This causes the nerves coming out of his spine and passing toward his arm to suddenly stretch or compress, which sends a burst of nerve messages streaming down the arm. The arm feels numb, weak, and tingly; and while the pain tends to go away soon, the weakness may persist for years. Protecting the arm, resting it, and using ice and compression for swelling and pain can help alleviate the condition. Most stingers heal by themselves.

Turf toe is an irritation of the joint at the base of the first or big toe. It usually happens when the toe is forcefully jammed against the ground or bent backward. The injury is more common in those playing on hard surfaces, such as artificial turf. The result is pain and swelling at the base of the toe, which hampers the athlete, especially when walking. The injury can be diagnosed by a physical exam and an X ray. The toe is usually treated without surgery, using ice, pain/anti-inflammatory medication, and elevation of the foot. If the patient has bone spurs and needs surgery, he likely will have to wear a cast. Wearing stiff-soled shoes and avoiding playing on artificial turf can help reduce the chances of getting this injury.

AIDS AND EXERCISE

According to the Centers for Disease Control and Prevention (CDC), more than 240,000 Americans are living with Acquired Immune Deficiency Syndrome (AIDS), a disease caused by a retrovirus, the human immunodeficiency virus (HIV). There is a growing body of evidence that exercise training can improve mood state and quality of life for HIV-positive individuals, and there is widespread belief among the HIV community that exercise training will make them stronger, improve their endurance, and protect them from infection. The symptoms of HIV infection vary during the course of the disease. In the first few months following infection with the virus, many people notice mononucleosislike symptoms. After that, the disease enters a symptom-free stage that may last up to ten to fifteen years. Eventually, as the infection takes its toll on the immune system, patients begin to experience night sweats and fevers, swollen glands, anorexia, and digestive complaints, widespread musculoskeletal aches and pains, and fatigue. This collection of symptoms is referred to as AIDS-related complex (ARC). AIDS, the most advanced stage of the disease, is diagnosed in HIV-infected people when CD4-positive cell counts become very low and opportunistic infections or cancers occur.

INTRODUCING EXERCISE

HIV infection can lead to loss of muscle strength and reduced aerobic capacity. Deconditioning often becomes more severe as the disease progresses. An appropriate program of exercise can improve exercise capacity in infected people and prevent or delay the downward spiral of deconditioning. Unfortunately, there is no evidence that exercise directly stimulates immune function or slows the onset of AIDS in HIV-infected people. However, regular exercise does have psychological benefits and can enhance the overall quality of life for HIV-positive people.

STARTING AN EXERCISE PROGRAM

Persons living with HIV/AIDS should consult their physician before beginning an exercise program or increasing their level of physical activity. A physician can offer advice on HIV-related medical conditions and side effects of medications that might affect one's ability to exercise.

An appropriate exercise program includes three basic components: aerobic exercise, strength training, and stretching activities to improve flexibility. In the early weeks of exercise training, sticking to light or moderate-intensity activity will improve physical conditioning without harming immune function. A plan might include exercising three to four times per week on alternate days and can include twenty minutes of light low-impact aerobic activity.

SEXUAL PROBLEMS

Sexual dysfunction refers to a problem during any phase of the sexual-response cycle that prevents the individual or couple from experiencing satisfaction from sexual activity. The sexual-response cycle has four phases: excitement, plateau, orgasm, and resolution.

While research suggests that sexual dysfunction is common (31 percent of men report some degree of difficulty), it is a topic that many people are hesitant to discuss. Fortunately, most cases of sexual dysfunction are treatable, so it is important to share your concerns with your partner and doctor.

WHAT CAUSES SEXUAL PROBLEMS?

Sexual dysfunction can be a result of a physical or psychological problem.

- **Physical causes:** Many physical and/or medical conditions can cause problems with sexual function. These conditions include diabetes, heart and vascular (blood vessel) disease, neurological disorders, hormonal imbalances, chronic diseases such as kidney or liver failure, and alcoholism or drug abuse. In addition, the side effects of certain medications, including some antidepressant drugs, can affect sexual desire and function.

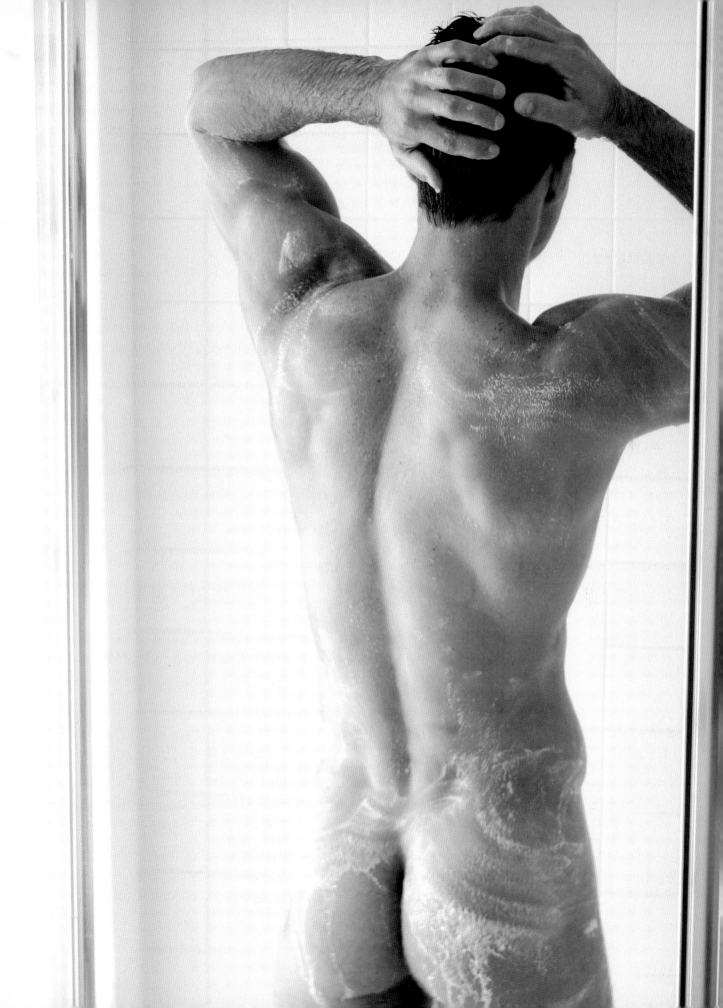

- Psychological causes: These include work-related stress and anxiety, concern about sexual performance, marital or relationship problems, depression, feelings of guilt, and the effects of a past sexual trauma.

WHO IS AFFECTED BY SEXUAL PROBLEMS?

Both men and women are affected by sexual problems. It is more common in the early adult years, with the majority of people seeking help during their late twenties and early thirties. Sexual dysfunction is also common in the geriatric population, which may be related to a decline in health associated with aging.

HOW DO SEXUAL PROBLEMS AFFECT MEN?

The most common sexual problems in men are ejaculation disorders, erectile dysfunction, and inhibited sexual desire.

WHAT ARE EJACULATION DISORDERS?

There are different types of ejaculation disorders, including:

- Premature ejaculation. This refers to ejaculation that occurs before or soon after penetration.

- Inhibited or retarded ejaculation. This is when ejaculation does not occur.

- Retrograde ejaculation. This occurs when, at orgasm, the ejaculate is forced back into the bladder rather than through the urethra and out the end of the penis.

In some cases, premature and inhibited ejaculation are caused by psychological factors, including a strict religious background that causes the person to view sex as sinful, a lack of attraction for a partner, and past traumatic events. Premature ejaculation, the most common form of sexual dysfunction in men, often is due to nervousness over how well he will perform during sex. Certain drugs, including some antidepressants, may affect ejaculation, as can nerve damage to the spinal cord or back.

Retrograde ejaculation is most common in males with diabetes who suffer from diabetic neuropathy (nerve damage). This is due to problems with the nerves in the bladder and the bladder neck that allow the ejaculate to flow backward. In other men, retrograde ejaculation occurs after operations on the bladder, neck, or prostate, or after certain abdominal operations. In addition, certain medications, particularly those used to treat mood disorders, may cause problems with ejaculation.

WHAT IS ERECTILE DYSFUNCTION?

Also known as impotence, erectile dysfunction is defined as the inability to attain and/or maintain an erection suitable for intercourse. Causes of erectile dysfunction include diseases affecting blood flow, such as atherosclerosis (hardening of the arteries); nerve disorders; psychological factors, such as stress, depression, and performance anxiety (nervousness over one's ability to sexually perform); and injury to the penis. Chronic illness, certain medications, and a condition called Peyronie's disease (scar tissue in the penis) also can cause erectile dysfunction.

WHAT IS INHIBITED SEXUAL DESIRE?

Inhibited desire, or loss of libido, refers to a decrease in desire for, or interest in sexual activity. Reduced libido can result from physical or psychological factors. It has been associated with low levels of the hormone testosterone. It also may be caused by psychological problems, such as anxiety and depression; medical illnesses, such as diabetes and high blood pressure; certain medications, including some antidepressants; and relationship difficulties.

HOW ARE MALE SEXUAL PROBLEMS DIAGNOSED?

The doctor likely will begin with a physical exam and a thorough history of symptoms. He or she may order other tests to rule out any medical problems that may be contributing to the dysfunction. The doctor may refer you to other doctors, including a urologist (a doctor specializing in the urinary tract and male reproductive system), an endocrinologist (a doctor specializing in glandular disorders), a neurologist (a doctor specializing in disorders of the nervous system), sex therapists, and other counselors.

WHAT TESTS ARE USED TO EVALUATE SEXUAL PROBLEMS?

- Blood tests. These tests are done to evaluate hormone levels.

- Vascular assessment. This involves an evaluation of the blood flow to the penis. A blockage in a blood vessel supplying blood to the penis may be contributing to erectile dysfunction.

- Sensory testing. Particularly useful in evaluating the effects of diabetic neuropathy (nerve damage), sensory testing measures the strength of nerve impulses in a particular area of the body.

- Nocturnal penile tumescence and rigidity testing. This test is used to monitor erections that occur naturally during sleep. This test can help determine if a man's erectile problems are due to physical or psychological causes.

HOW IS MALE SEXUAL DYSFUNCTION TREATED?

Many cases of sexual dysfunction can be corrected by treating the underlying physical or psychological problems. Treatment strategies may include the following:

- Medical treatment. This involves treatment of any physical problem that may be contributing to a man's sexual dysfunction.

- Medications. New medications, such as Viagra, may help improve sexual function in men by increasing blood flow to the penis.

- Hormones. Men with low levels of testosterone may benefit from hormone injections. The FDA has approved the use of a testosterone patch to raise testosterone levels to a normal range. Testosterone replacement by pills and implantable pellets also is being evaluated.

- Psychological therapy. Therapy with a trained counselor can help a person address feelings of anxiety, fear, or guilt that may have an impact on sexual function.

- Mechanical aids. Aids such as vacuum devices and penile implants may help men with erectile dysfunction.

- Education and communication. Education about sex and sexual behaviors and responses may help a man overcome his anxieties about sexual performance. Open dialogue

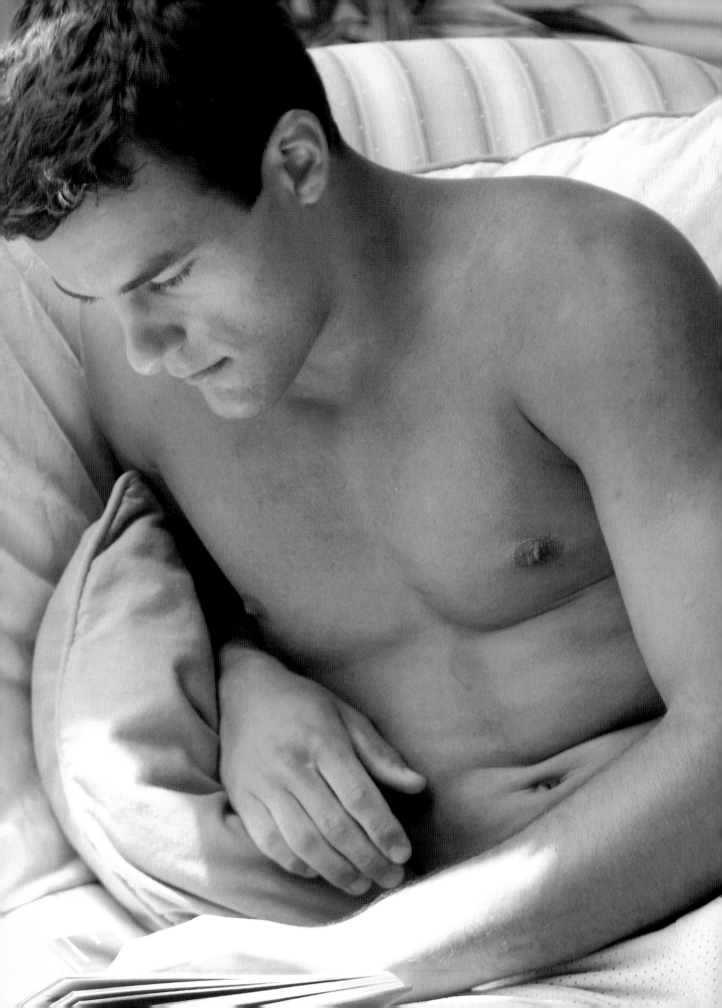

with your partner about your needs and concerns also helps to overcome many barriers to a healthy sex life.

CAN SEXUAL PROBLEMS BE CURED?

The success of treatment for sexual dysfunction depends on the underlying cause of the problem. The outlook is good for dysfunction that is related to a treatable or reversible physical condition. Mild dysfunction that is related to stress, fear, or anxiety often can be successfully treated with counseling, education, and improved communication between partners.

CAN SEXUAL PROBLEMS BE PREVENTED?

While sexual problems cannot be prevented, dealing with the underlying causes of the dysfunction can help you better understand and cope with the problem when it occurs. There are some things you can do to help maintain good sexual function:

- Limit alcohol intake.

- Follow your doctor's treatment plan for any medical/health conditions.

- Quit smoking.

- Deal with any emotional or psychological issues such as stress, depression, and anxiety. Get treatment as needed.

- Increase communication with your partner.

WHEN SHOULD I CALL MY DOCTOR?

Many men experience a problem with sexual function from time to time. However, when the problems are persistent, they can cause distress for the man and his partner and have a negative impact on their relationship. If you consistently experience sexual function problems, especially with erectile dysfunction, see your doctor for evaluation and treatment.

Masturbation is the self-stimulation of the genitals to achieve sexual arousal and pleasure, usually to the point of orgasm (sexual climax). It is commonly done by touching, stroking, or massaging the penis or clitoris until an orgasm is achieved. Some women also use stimulation of the vagina to masturbate or use "sex toys," such as a vibrator.

WHO MASTURBATES?

Just about everybody. Masturbation is a very common behavior, even among people who have sexual relations with a partner. In one national study, 95 percent of males and 89 percent of females reported that they have masturbated. Masturbation is the first sexual act experienced by most males and females. In children, masturbation is a normal part of exploring his or her body. Most people continue to masturbate in adulthood, and many do so throughout their lives.

WHY DO PEOPLE MASTURBATE?

In addition to feeling good, masturbation is a way of relieving the sexual tension that can build up over time, especially for people without partners or whose partners are not willing or available for sex. When sexual dysfunction is present in an adult, masturbation may be prescribed by a sex therapist to allow a person to experience an orgasm (often in women) or to delay its arrival (often in men).

The only behavior that I WILL get really militant about in this book is smoking cigarettes. As an ex-smoker (two packs a day for over fifteen years), I know we are the worst converts. It just pains me to see people who train hard physically and work so hard at keeping fit doing the one thing that is completely against every principle they are working so hard to achieve. Smoking is the number-one preventable cause of death in America. It was back in 1964 that the surgeon general presented scientific evidence on the hazards of smoking. Today it is believed to be even worse for your health—not only for the smoker, but for the people around them as well.

If the cancer risk is not enough to scare you, consider that heart attacks are twice as likely to happen to the smoker than the nonsmoker. The World Health Organization (WHO) stated that controlling cigarette smoking could do more to improve the health and prolong life in developed countries than any single action in the entire field of preventative medicine. Doesn't that tell you something?

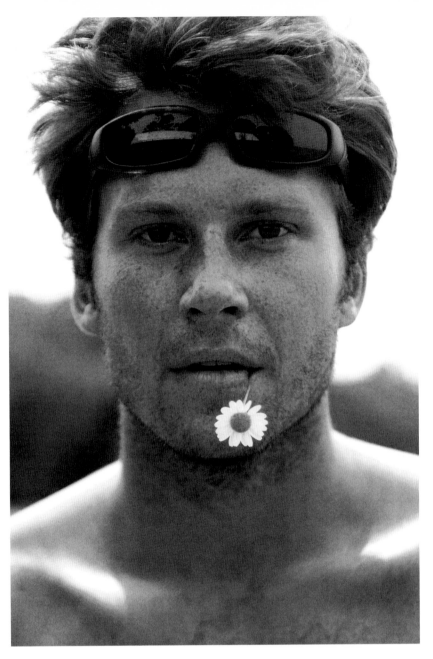

STOP—YOU CAN!

By quitting now, you can reduce the risk of having a heart attack to the same level as a nonsmoker in just a few months. Your lungs are pretty remarkable this way. The act like sponges and have the ability to cleanse themselves over time. There may be damage that cannot be undone, but one of the major causes of heart disease will be removed. More people succumb to heart disease each year than lung cancer. Tightness in the chest should relax after only a few weeks.

WITHDRAWAL FROM THE BIG N

Nicotine is what a smoker's body craves. The body adapts to the level of nicotine that you deliver with each cigarette. When you take the agent away, the body will react in a variety of ways, such as intense mood swings and physical changes. Some of the side effects may be as follows:

Irritability

Nervousness

Exhaustion

Hunger

Dry mouth

HOW TO GET OVER SOME OF THE SIDE EFFECTS

IRRITABILITY. This will subside with time. Patience will be the real antidote. Having friends who understand what you are going through will also serve as a safety net.

NERVOUSNESS. Find something to occupy your hands and head—a hobby, puzzles, worry balls, meditation exercises, a yoga class.

EXHAUSTION. Aerobic exercise will give you a boost. Eight hours of sleep will also help you in the detoxification period.

HUNGER. Stay away from sweets if you can and have a container of celery sticks around at all times.

DRY MOUTH. Water will help you filter the nicotine out of your system, and sugarless gum might help you with the dry mouth.

There are many methods to support your effort to quit: gums, patches, hypnosis, and acupuncture to name a few. What worked for me? I tried them all, but until I understood my behavior, I was never successful. In fact, I would leave my acupuncturist and smoke because I felt so relaxed. I went to the American Heart Association Smoke Enders program, where they hold a mirror up to your habit. They asked us to do a simple exercise in understanding our habit. We were instructed to wrap a pack of cigarettes with a piece of paper. Each and every time we smoked, we had to unwrap the pack, write down the time of day and how we felt— without exception. Not only was it a pain in the rear to unwrap the pack every time, the ritual was embarrassing in front of people, and all in all it was annoying. Each time the group met, which was once a week, we had to share with each other how many butts we had smoked and read what feelings were most common.

What this exercise was able to point out to all of us was the behavior around the nicotine habit. I used cigarettes to tell stories, drink coffee, after sex, on the phone, after dinner, and walking around the city. I spent a lot of time smoking. When I saw how much time I was wasting, I was embarrassed. I knew I could use that time more efficiently. I had that long-awaited epiphany. I quit cold turkey. It just happened one day when I decided to grow up and get rid of this ugly habit. There, that is all I have to say about that without creating too many enemies. Think it through before you continue to smoke. It really isn't that cool, it costs a small fortune in most places, and you will breathe easier without the habit.

BRING IT ON—LATER: ANTIAGING TOOLS

EAT A GOOD BREAKFAST EVERY DAY.

- Use fruits, milk, yogurt, hot or cold cereal, low-fat cheeses, and instant breakfast mixes.

- Try low-fat milk and a bran flake–type cereal. You get calcium, B-complex vitamins, and fiber (5.5 grams in two cups).

GET ENOUGH PROTEIN.

- Rotate skinless chicken, fish, and lean meats as main courses.

- Have daily doses of whole grains, nuts, seeds, peas, and dry beans.

- Use low- or nonfat dairy products regularly.

- Eat eggs occasionally.

DRINK PLENTY OF WATER.

- Water makes up more than half your body composition and must be replaced daily.

- You need it to regulate body temperature, digest foods, and prevent constipation.

- Drinking coffee, tea, and alcohol increases water loss (try cocoa instead).

- Popsicles and fruit juices are good alternatives to plain water.

- Exercise increases the need for water.

FIBER IS IMPORTANT.

- It aids digestion, prevents constipation, and decreases cholesterol, and blood sugar.

- Eat whole grain cereals.

- Eat vegetables (and fruits), raw when possible with skin.

- Add dry beans to soups, stews, and salads.

MINIMIZE HIGH SUGAR AND PROCESSED FOODS.

- Sweets and desserts tend to be high in calories and low in nutrients.

- Soda pops and other sugared drinks are poor beverage choices (try water or pure fruit juice instead).

- Minimize the use of table sugar and syrups.

CHAPTER TWELVE

RESOURCE GUIDE

Following are some companies that have always been helpful to me and have shown compassion to the rest of the world.

HELPFUL COMPANIES

ACSM

401 West Michigan Street

Indianapolis, IN 46202-3233

MAILING ADDRESS

P.O. Box 1440

Indianapolis, IN 46206-1440

Telephone 1-317-637-9200 or 1-317-637-9200, ext. 138

Fax 1-317-634-7817

www.acsm.org

Great information Source

DYNAMIX MUSIC INC.

9411 Philadelphia Road, Baltimore, MD 21237

Office Hours: Mon.–Fri., 9 A.M.–9 P.M., Sat. 9 A.M.–5 P.M. EST

1-800-843-6499 or 1-410-918-1000

Fax 1-410-918-1863

Music Preview Line 1-410-918-9518

www.dynamixmusic.com

Workout Music for All Acivities

NAUTILUS HEALTH AND FITNESS GROUP

1886 Prairie Way

Louisville, CO 80027

Telephone 303-939-0100

www.nautilusgroup.com

Nautilus Strength Equipment, Scwhinn, Stairmaster, Boloflex Products

POLAR HEART RATE MONITORS

Polar Electro Inc.

370 Crossways Park Drive

Woodbury, NY 11797-2050

Telephone 1-800-227-1314

Fax 1-516-364-5454

www.polarusa.com

Heartrate Monitors

POWER SYSTEM INC.

P.O. Box 31709

Knoxville, TN 37930

Telephone 1-800-321-6975 toll free anytime 24-hours a day (or dial direct 1-865-769-8223)

Fax 1-800-298-2057 toll free anytime 24-hours a day (or direct 1-865-769-8211)

Stability Balls, Medicine Balls, Mats, Weights

MEDICINE BALL EXERCISES AT A GLANCE

YOGA-INSPIRED EXERCISES AT A GLANCE

Q & A

Q: *I lost forty pounds and I'm worried I'm going to gain it all back because I'm constantly hungry. Is there anything I can do?*

A: This question is at the heart of losing and most importantly, maintaining weight. That's because weight loss is relatively easy in the short term as it only requires enough willpower to deny yourself food for a short time. But typically, you eventually give in and overcompensate for the calories that you've been denying yourself. The result: Weight regain. So any tricks to prevent hunger from getting the better of you can be very valuable.

Including a little protein with each meal or snack can help suppress your hunger. That's because protein has the strongest effect on reducing appetite, compared to carbohydrates and fat. Drinking water may alleviate hunger as well since it can make you feel full. Plus, by sipping on water all day long, you'll be less likely to reach for calories—drinks like juices and soft drinks. And, of course, eating high-fiber foods such as fruit, vegetables, and whole grains can give you the feeling of being full without adding too many calories. Try to consciously incorporate each of these three

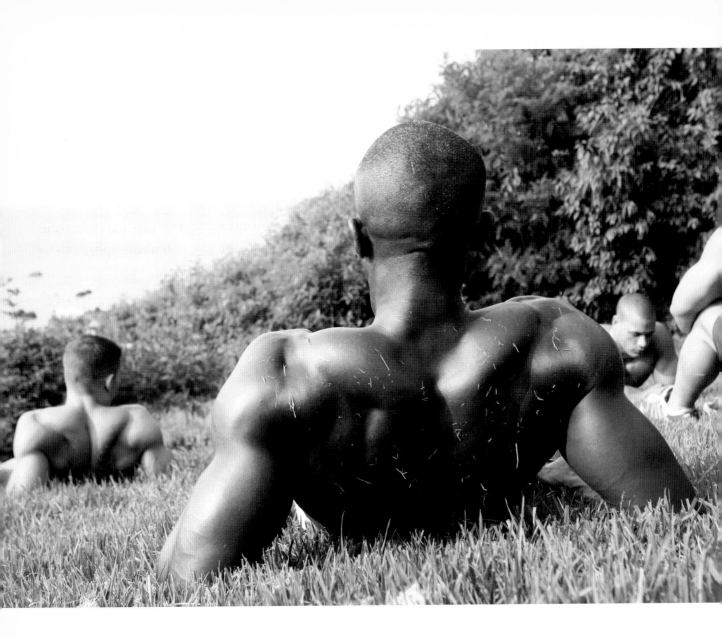

things into each meal and snack, and you should be able to eat a reduced-calorie diet without as much hunger.

Q: *My main goal is to lose fat. Will three full-body workouts a week (every other day) be just as effective as a four-day routine in which I work a split routine twice?*

A: In my opinion, three full-body workouts will be more effective, assuming your total training volume is similar. That's because you'll work more total muscle fibers each workout, which will cause your body to burn more calories both during and after each exercise session. Plus, by their nature, full-body workouts are simply harder than lower-body- or upper-body-only workouts.

So if overall fat loss is your primary objective, total body training is a far superior system than splitting up body parts. I'd recommend doing three full-body workouts a week, but with different exercises each day. That is, don't do regular squats three days a week. Instead, maybe do front squats one day, dead lifts on day two, and regular squats on day three. It'll increase the variety in your workout and ensure you're working your entire body equally.

Q: *How much body fat can I expect to lose a week if I'm working out regularly and following a strict diet?*

A: Typically, a good training program should result in about 0.5 percent of body fat per week, and a good diet should result in the same. So ideally, you should shoot for a body-fat loss of about 1 percent a week. That's the goal I use with my clients. The key is to monitor your results weekly so that you can make changes—reduce or increase your caloric intake, increase your physical activity, get more rest—if you're not achieving fat loss at that rate. Remember, these are the ideal results under consistent application of an appropriate nutrition plan and intense training program.

Q: *I have read numerous articles weighing the weight-loss benefits of aerobic training versus weight lifting. What's the best way?*

A: Research shows that aerobic exercise burns more calories and fat during exercise than weight lifting. However, there is strong evidence that shows weight lifting burns more calories and fat for a longer period of time after exercise. From a physiological perspective, you have to appreciate that aerobic exercise and weight lifting are doing two very different things to the body. Generally speaking, aerobic exercise has favorable effects on your cardiorespiratory system (your heart, lungs, and blood vessels) whereas weight lifting has favorable effects on skeletal muscle. That is, it increases the size and strength of your muscles. Studies that have examined weight-loss programs that involve diet only, diet plus aerobic exercise, or diet plus aerobic exercise and weight lifting show some interesting results. Generally speaking, these studies report that dieting alone results in about the same weight loss as diet plus exercise. However, more fat is lost and muscle preserved if you add aerobic exercise. And even more fat is lost and muscle preserved if you add aerobic exercise *and* weight lifting.

Do the one you like the best, since you're most likely to stick with it. If you don't have a preference, go with weight lifting. You may not lose weight as fast as with aerobic exercise, but you'll lose just as much fat, while maintaining more of your muscle.

Throughout this book I have tried to inspire the importance of balance not only in your life, but also in your body. Remember, 50 percent of success is trying; the other 50 percent is practice. Balance will find you. Be patient, be consistent, be commited.